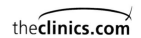

GASTROENTEROLOGY CLINICS OF NORTH AMERICA

Gastrointestinal Bleeding

GUEST EDITOR
Don C. Rockey, MD

December 2005 • Volume 34 • Number 4

SAUNDERS
An Imprint of Elsevier, Inc.
PHILADELPHIA   LONDON   TORONTO   MONTREAL   SYDNEY   TOKYO

W.B. SAUNDERS COMPANY
A Division of Elsevier Inc.

Elsevier Inc. • 1600 John F. Kennedy Blvd., Suite 1800 • Philadelphia, Pennsylvania 19103-2899

http://www.theclinics.com

GASTROENTEROLOGY CLINICS
OF NORTH AMERICA   Volume 34, Number 4
December 2005   ISSN 0889-8553
Editor: Kerry Holland   ISBN 1-4160-2785-8

The ideas and opinions expressed in *Gastroenterology Clinics of North America* do not necessarily reflect those of the Publisher. The Publisher does not assume any responsibility for any injury and/or damage to persons or property arising out of or related to any use of the material contained in this periodical. The reader is advised to check the appropriate medical literature and the product information currently provided by the manufacturer of each drug to be administered to verify the dosage, the method and duration of administration, or contraindications. It is the responsibility of the treating physician or other health care professional, relying on independent experience and knowledge of the patient, to determine drug dosages and the best treatment for the patient. Mention of any product in this issue should not be construed as endorsement by the contributors, editors, or the Publisher of the product or manufacturers' claims.

Gastroenterology Clinics of North America (ISSN 0889-8553) is published quarterly by W.B. Saunders Company. Corporate and Editorial Offices: Elsevier Inc., 1600 John F. Kennedy Blvd., Suite 1800, Philadelphia, PA 19103-2899. Accounting and Circulation Offices: 6277 Sea Harbor Drive, Orlando, FL 32887-4800. Periodicals postage paid at Orlando, FL 32862, and additional mailing offices. Subscription prices are $195.00 per year (US individuals), $100.00 per year (US students), $290.00 per year (US institutions), $215.00 per year (Canadian individuals), $345.00 per year (Canadian institutions), $255.00 per year (international individuals), $130.00 per year (international students), and $345.00 per year (international institutions). Foreign air speed delivery is included in all *Clinics* subscription prices. All prices are subject to change without notice. POSTMASTER: Send address changes to *Gastroenterology Clinics of North America*, W.B. Saunders Company, Periodicals Fulfillment, Orlando, FL 32887-4800. **Customer Service: 1-800-654-2452 (US). From outside of the US, call 1-407-345-4000. E-mail: hhspcs@harcourt.com**

Gastroenterology Clinics of North America is also published in Italian by Il Pensiero Scientifico Editore, Rome, Italy; and in Portuguese by Interlivros Edicoes Ltda., Rua Commandante Coelho 1085, 21250 Cordovil, Rio de Janeiro, Brazil.

Gastroenterology Clinics of North America is covered in *Index Medicus, Excerpta Medica, Current Contents/ Clinical Medicine, Science Citation Index, ISI/BIOMED*, and *BIOSIS*.

Printed in the United States of America.

GASTROENTEROLOGY CLINICS
OF NORTH AMERICA

Gastrointestinal Bleeding

GUEST EDITOR

DON C. ROCKEY, MD, Professor of Medicine; Chief, Division of Digestive and Liver Diseases, University of Texas Southwestern Medical Center, Dallas, Texas

CONTRIBUTORS

ELIZABETH J. CAREY, MD, Assistant Professor of Medicine, Gastroenterology and Hepatology, Mayo Clinic, Scottsdale, Arizona

NAGA CHALASANI, MD, Associate Professor of Medicine, Indiana University School of Medicine, Indianapolis, Indiana

ERIC ESRAILIAN, MD, Division of Digestive Diseases, David Geffen School of Medicine at UCLA, UCLA/VA Center for Outcomes Research and Education, Los Angeles, California

CHARLES B FERGUSON, MB, MRCP, Gastroenterology Fellow, Department of Gastroenterology, Belfast City Hospital, Belfast, Northern Ireland

DAVID E. FLEISCHER, MD, Professor of Medicine, Gastroenterology and Hepatology, Mayo Clinic, Scottsdale, Arizona

IAN M. GRALNEK, MD, MSHS, Technion Faculty of Medicine, Department of Gastroenterology, Rambam Medical Center, Haifa, Israel; Formerly, Associate Professor of Medicine, David Geffen School of Medicine at UCLA, VA Greater Los Angeles Healthcare System, Center for the Study of Digestive Healthcare Quality and Outcomes, Los Angeles, California

BRYAN T. GREEN, MD, Digestive Diseases Group, Greenwood, South Carolina; Formerly, Division of Gastroenterology, Department of Medicine, Duke University Medical Center, Durham, North Carolina

SAUYU LIN, MD, Trinity Clinic, Tyler, Texas; Formerly, Division of Gastroenterology, Duke University Medical Center, Durham, North Carolina

MICHAEL MILLER, Jr, MD, Associate, Department of Radiology, Duke University Medical Center, Durham, North Carolina

ROBERT M. MITCHELL, MB, MRCP, Consultant Gastroenterologist, Department of Gastroenterology, Belfast City Hospital, Belfast, Northern Ireland

DON C. ROCKEY, MD, Professor of Medicine; Chief, Division of Digestive and Liver Diseases, University of Texas Southwestern Medical Center, Dallas, Texas

TONY P. SMITH, MD, Professor, Department of Radiology, Duke University Medical Center, Durham, North Carolina

LISA L. STRATE, MD, MPH, Instructor in Medicine, Harvard Medical School; Division of Gastroenterology, Brigham and Women's Hospital, Boston, Massachusetts

ATIF ZAMAN, MD, MPH, Associate Professor of Medicine, Oregon Health Sciences University, Portland, Oregon

GASTROENTEROLOGY CLINICS
OF NORTH AMERICA

Gastrointestinal Bleeding

CONTENTS

VOLUME 34 • NUMBER 4 • DECEMBER 2005

> Gastrointestinal bleeding encompasses a broad array of clinical scenarios. The spectrum is diverse because of the multiple types of lesions that can cause bleeding, and because bleeding can occur from virtually anywhere in the gastrointestinal tract. The fundamental tenets of management of patients with gastrointestinal bleeding include the following: (1) the patient must undergo immediate assessment and stabilization of hemodynamic status, (2) the source of bleeding must be identified, (3) active bleeding should be stopped, (4) the underlying abnormality should be treated, and (5) recurrent bleeding should be prevented.

> Nonvariceal upper gastrointestinal bleeding remains an important cause of patient morbidity, mortality, and use of considerable health care resources. An early and accurate diagnosis is critical for guiding appropriate management and facilitating patient care. This article reviews the most recent epidemiologic data on acute nonvariceal upper gastrointestinal bleeding and outlines important aspects of making the diagnosis.

> Nonvariceal upper gastrointestinal bleeding remains a challenging problem with a significant morbidity and mortality. In recent years endoscopic techniques have evolved, resulting in improved primary hemostasis and a reduction in the risk of rebleeding. Combination endoscopic therapy followed by high-dose proton pump inhibitor shows improved outcomes. Innovative endoscopic therapies hold promise but are as yet unproved. An aging population with significant medical comorbidities has a major influence on the overall outcome from upper gastrointestinal bleeding.

Occult gastrointestinal (GI) bleeding is the most common form of GI bleeding, and it takes the form of two important clinical scenarios, namely fecal occult blood or iron deficiency anemia. Evidence suggests that in men and postmenopausal women who have iron deficiency anemia, GI tract pathology is the source for blood loss. As such, evaluation of patients with iron deficiency anemia generally focuses on the GI tract. It is critical that the diagnosis of iron deficiency anemia be established firmly before extensive evaluation is undertaken. Fecal occult blood loss is even more common than iron deficiency anemia. Management strategies for patients with fecal occult blood/iron deficiency anemia are reviewed; an important general point is that clinical features (ie, symptoms) may help direct specific investigation. The role of small intestinal investigation in patients with fecal occult blood/iron deficiency anemia is controversial, and probably should be reserved for patients who have iron deficiency anemia and persistent GI symptoms or those who fail to respond to appropriate therapy. Treatment and prognosis of patients with fecal occult blood/iron deficiency anemia depend on the underlying cause of blood loss.

Small intestinal bleeding presents a unique clinical problem that differs from upper and lower gastrointestinal (GI) bleeding in many respects. Patients who have small intestinal bleeding undergo more diagnostic procedures, require more blood transfusions, have longer hospitalizations, and have higher health care expenditures than patients who have upper or lower GI bleeding. The difficulty accessing the small bowel endoscopically may contribute to this phenomenon. This article reviews pertinent enteroscopy techniques, with an emphasis on the new technologies of capsule endoscopy and double balloon enteroscopy.

The angiographic evaluation of non variceal gastrointestinal (GI) hemorrhage has been used for years. In the upper GI tract its diagnostic role is limited; however, intervention with embolization has become the preferred treatment in cases of failure to control bleeding through endoscopic intervention. In the lower GI tract the diagnostic and therapeutic value of angiography has been chosen in most institutions as the primary modality for controlling bleeding. The choice of vasopressin verses embolization has been studied in many case reviews. The movement toward embolotherapy and its implications on clinical resolution of bleeding and ischemia will be discussed. Our goal is to bring a synopsis of the literature into a format which will help clarify the interventionist's view of the endovascular options to control GI bleeding.

GASTROENTEROLOGY CLINICS
OF NORTH AMERICA

ELSEVIER
SAUNDERS

Gastroenterol Clin N Am 34 (2005) xi–xiii

GASTROENTEROLOGY CLINICS
OF NORTH AMERICA

PREFACE

Gastrointestinal Bleeding

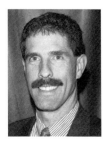

Don C. Rockey, MD
Guest Editor

Gastrointestinal bleeding is one of the most common clinical problems in all of medicine and in gastroenterology. Gastrointestinal bleeding can be accompanied by any of a number of clinical presentations. The most common source of overt gastrointestinal bleeding is the upper gastrointestinal tract, whereas bleeding from small bowel or colon is important, but a less common source. Bleeding from the small intestine is particularly challenging. Obscure and occult gastrointestinal bleeding occurs as a result of gastrointestinal tract abnormalities in any region of the gut (or, on occasion, organs linked to the gut). Occult gastrointestinal bleeding may be clinically evident or hidden altogether. If the bleeding site remains unknown after routine endoscopic evaluation, but is clinically evident, the bleeding is coined obscure bleeding. Bleeding that is hidden completely is typically designated occult bleeding.

The current edition, devoted in its entirety to gastrointestinal bleeding, begins with presentation of a practical approach to managing gastrointestinal bleeding. The edition next turns to upper gastrointestinal bleeding. This common and important cause of gastrointestinal bleeding can be caused by an abnormality in the esophagus, stomach, or proximal small bowel. A wealth of data on this topic has been published, and its review begins with a discussion of the epidemiology and diagnosis of upper gastrointestinal bleeding by Drs. Eric Esrailian and Ian Gralneck. They review the most recent epidemiologic data on acute nonvariceal upper gastrointestinal bleeding and outline critical aspects of making an appropriate diagnosis.

0889-8553/05/$ – see front matter
doi:10.1016/j.gtc.2005.08.001

Next, Drs. Charlie Ferguson and Mike Mitchell review the treatment of non-varical upper gastrointestinal bleeding. This topic, more than any other, has set the standard for management in the field of gastrointestinal bleeding. For example, data now clearly demonstrate that endoscopic intervention reduces rebleeding and mortality in patients with high-risk ulcer lesions. Newer data suggests that pharmacologic intervention (with proton-pump inhibitors) also reduces the risk of rebleeding. Finally, a number of newer endoscopic therapeutic approaches are being introduced in the area of upper gastrointestinal bleeding, and these are reviewed.

One of the most feared complications of cirrhosis and portal hypertension is variceal hemorrhage. Usually due to esophageal variceal rupture, this complication occurs in an entirely different epidemiologic and clinical setting than nonvariceal upper gastrointestinal bleeding. Thus, this topic, reviewed by Drs. Atif Zaman and Naga Chalasani, requires understanding of many critical issues, including diagnosis and management. Drs. Zaman and Chalasani have elegantly reviewed all critical issues in this area, including those related to management of acute bleeding, prevention of recurrent bleeding, and prevention of the first variceal bleed.

The issue next turns to the topic of lower gastrointestinal bleeding. Lower gastrointestinal bleeding differs from upper gastrointestinal bleeding in many ways. First, the epidemiology of lower gastrointestinal bleeding is substantially different than that of upper gastrointestinal bleeding. Additionally, the diagnostic approach to lower gastrointestinal bleeding is considerably different than that for upper gastrointestinal bleeding. Therefore, the epidemiology and diagnosis of lower gastrointestinal bleeding are first reviewed by one of the leading authorities in this area, Dr. Lisa Strate. The management of lower gastrointestinal bleeding is evolving. Historically, various approaches have been undertaken. A common approach has been watchful waiting, often with elective colonoscopy being performed after bleeding has subsided. However, it remains distinctly possible that more aggressive intervention could lead to improved outcomes. Dr. Byran Green has reviewed the state of the art with regard to management approaches for lower gastrointestinal bleeding, including the usefulness of urgent colonoscopy.

Patients with obscure gastrointestinal bleeding present perhaps the most challenging problems in all patients with gastrointestinal bleeding. This is because by definition they have had multiple episodes of bleeding and have therefore been previously evaluated without identification of a definitive bleeding site. Perhaps the most critical issue on the topic of obscure GI bleeding is that intervention be tailored to each individual based on specific patient characteristics. Thus, Dr. Sauyu Lin reviewed many critical issues on this subject with emphasis on the role of enteroscopy, other diagnostic approaches, and management.

I have included a review on true occult gastrointestinal bleeding, including iron-deficiency anemia and fecal occult blood. This type of bleeding, though rarely life threatening, is perhaps the most common form of gastrointestinal bleeding. It has substantial overlap with the other forms of gastrointestinal bleeding and requires a thoughtful and focused approach.

One of the most exciting advances in gastrointestinal endoscopy has been the recent introduction of capsule endoscopy, which has become a favored diagnostic tool in various types of patients with gastrointestinal bleeding. This technique, along with enteroscopy, has gained extraordinary momentum over the past several years as a tool to evaluate the small bowel. The issue of small bowel investigation and the use of enteroscopy and capsule endoscopy, is reviewed elegantly by Drs. Elizabeth Carey and David Fleischer.

Radiology and, in particular, interventional radiologic approaches have evolved substantially over the past decade, such that a number of effective and valuable tools for patients who have gastrointestinal bleeding are available. Indeed, interventional techniques have become a cornerstone in the management of many forms of gastrointestinal bleeding and are reviewed in detail by Drs. Michael Miller and Tony Smith. It is critical for the practitioner to be familiar with the radiographic techniques they have reviewed.

I am grateful to all of the authors who so willingly contributed to this issue, which is intentionally comprehensive in nature. I hope that you will find this issue as informative and helpful in your practice of medicine as I have.

Don C. Rockey, MD
Division of Digestive and Liver Diseases
University of Texas Southwestern Medical Center
5323 Harry Hines Boulevard
Dallas, TX 75390-8887, USA

E-mail address: don.rockey@utsouthwestern.edu

Gastroenterol Clin N Am 34 (2005) 581–588

GASTROENTEROLOGY CLINICS
OF NORTH AMERICA

Gastrointestinal Bleeding

Don C. Rockey, MD

Division of Digestive and Liver Diseases, University of Texas Southwestern Medical Center,
5323 Harry Hines Boulevard, Dallas, TX 75390–8887, USA

Gastrointestinal bleeding encompasses a broad array of clinical scenarios. The spectrum is diverse because of the multiple types of lesions that can cause bleeding, and because bleeding can occur from virtually anywhere in the gastrointestinal tract. Additionally, gastrointestinal bleeding varies greatly in its volume and as such may be massive or trivial, and may be clinically apparent or altogether hidden. Gastrointestinal bleeding is manifest in one or more of the following clinical scenarios: (1) bleeding is from the upper gastrointestinal tract; (2) bleeding is from the lower gastrointestinal tract; (3) bleeding is occult (ie, unknown to the patient); or (4) bleeding is clinically obvious but the site (ie, whether it is from the upper or lower gastrointestinal tract) is obscure. Patients with occult bleeding are challenging because the patient is unaware of the bleeding and clinical clues to its cause are typically lacking. Patients with obscure bleeding are particularly challenging because their bleeding is typically recurrent and the site of bleeding is difficult accurately to identify.

Gastrointestinal bleeding results in over 300,000 hospitalizations annually in the United States [1]. Bleeding from the upper gastrointestinal tract is approximately five times more common than from the lower gastrointestinal tract [2,3] and seems to be more common in men and the elderly [2,3].

Despite a number of recent advances in the management of patients with gastrointestinal bleeding, several fundamental clinical principles remain constant, the most important of which is immediate assessment and stabilization of the patient's hemodynamic status. Thereafter, a careful history and physical examination follows, and with it the etiology and source of bleeding predicted. Specific investigation then follows and further delineates the source of bleeding. Once the bleeding site is identified, it must be stopped and treated. Subsequently, recurrent bleeding should be prevented.

CLINICAL PRESENTATION

The clinical presentation of patients with gastrointestinal bleeding typically reflects the site, etiology, and rate of bleeding. Gastrointestinal tract bleeding is

E-mail address: don.rockey@utsouthwestern.edu

0889-8553/05/$ – see front matter
doi:10.1016/j.gtc.2005.08.002

manifest in one or more ways. Hematemesis, melena, or hematochezia are the most common manifestations of gastrointestinal bleeding. Hematemesis is defined as vomiting of blood and is caused by upper gastrointestinal bleeding from the esophagus, stomach, or proximal small bowel. Blood may be bright red or it may be old and take on the appearance of coffee grounds. Melena is defined as passage of black, tarry, and foul-smelling stools. The black, tarry character of melena is caused by degradation of blood in the more proximal colon (and is typical of bleeding from the upper gastrointestinal tract). Melena should not be confused with the greenish character of ingested iron or the black, non–foul-smelling stool caused by ingestion of bismuth (ie, in compounds, such as bismuth subsalicylate). Hematochezia refers to bright red blood from the rectum that may or may not be mixed with stool. Occult gastrointestinal bleeding denotes bleeding that is not apparent to the patient and is caused by small amounts of bleeding. Obscure gastrointestinal bleeding refers to obvious (eg, manifest by hematemesis, melena, or hematochezia) bleeding, but from a source that is not easily identified on routine examination.

INITIAL PATIENT ASSESSMENT

When a patient is found to have one of the previously mentioned manifestations of gastrointestinal bleeding, the first step in management should be to assess the severity of bleeding. Assessment of the patient's hemodynamics should be emphasized (Table 1). This hemodynamic assessment forms the basis for further management. Ongoing assessment of the vital signs further focuses resuscitation efforts, and also provides important prognostic information. Finally, ongoing and careful assessment of the patient's hemodynamic status helps triage appropriate intervention. For example, patients with obviously unstable vital signs are often bleeding from major vascular sources, such as an ulcer with a visible vessel or gastroesophageal varices; the prognosis of these patients is poorer than that of those with normal vital signs, and their clinical condition mandates more aggressive and timely intervention than patients with normal vital signs.

RESUSCITATION

The more severe the bleeding (ie, unstable vital signs and evidence of ongoing bleeding), the more vigorous the resuscitation efforts should be. In patients who have any evidence of hemodynamic instability, two large-bore intravenous

Table 1
Hemodynamics, vital signs, and blood loss

Hemodynamics vital sign	% Blood loss (fraction of intravascular volume)	Bleed type
Shock (resting hypotension)	20–25	Massive
Postural (orthostatic tachycardia or hypotension)	10–20	Moderate
Normal	<10	Minor

catheters should be placed immediately. Colloid (normal saline or lactated Ringer's solution) should be infused as rapidly as the patient's cardiovascular system allows to restore the vital signs toward normal. ICU monitoring is indicated in hemodynamically unstable patients. Supplemental oxygen by nasal cannula or facemask should be given liberally. Vital signs and urine output should be monitored closely, and in selected situations (for patients with underlying cardiopulmonary disease) central venous monitoring is helpful. The importance of aggressive ICU monitoring and resuscitation has been emphasized by investigation suggesting that it may decrease mortality [4].

In addition to colloidal solutions, patients must typically undergo blood transfusion. Decisions about when and how much to transfuse the patient with gastrointestinal bleeding is often complicated and requires integrations of multiple aspects of the clinical situation. Virtually all patients with unstable vital signs have had significant blood loss and require blood transfusion. If the patient has subnormal tissue oxygenation, transfusion should be aggressive. Patients with continued instability in vital signs, continued bleeding, symptoms of poor tissue oxygenation, or persistently low hematocrit values (20%–25%) likewise should probably be transfused continuously. It is most appropriate to raise the hematocrit to a level of 30% in elderly patients, whereas in younger, otherwise healthy patients, hematocrit values in the 20% to 25% range may be satisfactory; in those with portal hypertension, it should not be above 27% to 28%. Transfusion should be with packed red blood cells, except in rare circumstances where whole blood transfusions may be used in those who cannot be cross-matched in a timely fashion. In those with specific defects in coagulation factors or platelets, these substances can be replaced. Patients requiring greater than 10 units of packed red blood cells should receive fresh-frozen plasma or platelets or both. Warmed blood should be administered to patients requiring massive transfusions (ie, >3000 mL). The hematocrit should be monitored serially (typically after a specific transfusion). Serial hematocrits are not a substitute, however, for ongoing clinical assessment of the hemodynamics. Frequently, patients with chronic bleeding may have a low hematocrit, but no evidence of hemodynamic instability. In this situation, blood transfusion should be slow and deliberate, regardless of the hematocrit value.

HISTORY, SYMPTOMS, AND SIGNS

Once the patient's hemodynamics and overall condition has been assessed and stabilized, attention should turn to the clinical history. The history helps the clinician assess the severity of bleeding and make a preliminary assessment of the site and cause. Historical features important in assessing the etiology of gastrointestinal bleeding are shown in Box 1.

Simple demographic characteristics are an essential part of the history. For example, elderly patients may bleed from a number of diseases less common in younger persons (ie, vascular ectasia, diverticula, ischemic colitis, cancer), whereas bleeding in younger patients is more likely to be from esophagitis, varices, or Meckel's diverticula (typically lower gastrointestinal bleeding in

Box 1: Historical features in the assessment of gastrointestinal bleeding

Age
Prior bleeding
Previous gastrointestinal disease
Previous surgery
Underlying medical disorder (especially liver disease)
Nonsteroidal anti-inflammatory drugs (NSAIDs), aspirin (ASA)
Abdominal pain
Change in bowel habits
Weight loss or anorexia
History of oropharyngeal disease

patients under 30 years of age). A past history of previous gastrointestinal disease or previous bleeding should focus the differential diagnosis immediately on related bleeding (eg, hereditary hemorrhagic telangiectasia, ulcer disease, diverticular bleeding). A history of previous surgery is likewise important. For example, a history of previous aortic surgery should increase the suspicion for aortoenteric fistula. A history of liver disease raises the possibility of bleeding associated with portal hypertension. Ingestion of medications, such as aspirin or other nonsteroidal anti-inflammatory drugs, makes bleeding from ulceration more likely. Patients taking anticoagulant medications may be more likely to bleed from ulcers or vascular ectasias. Gastrointestinal bleeding in the setting of anticoagulation therapy, even in patients taking warfarin and who have a supratherapeutic international normalized ratio, is most often caused by underlying gastrointestinal tract pathology [5] and should not be ascribed to overanticoagulation. Other important historical features include abdominal pain (which suggests peptic ulcer disease, mesenteric or colonic ischemia); retching (Mallory-Weiss tear); or change in bowel habits, anorexia, or weight loss, all of which point to malignancy. Interestingly, elderly patients may be less likely to report abdominal pain associated with bleeding ulcers [6]. The history is also critical in ascertaining whether nongastrointestinal sources may be the cause of reported or witnessed bleeding, especially from the lungs or nasopharynx.

Physical examination should focus on putative evidence of liver disease (splenomegaly, ascites, caput), which increases the likelihood of portal hypertension and related causes of bleeding. The skin may also reveal evidence of chronic liver disease (eg, cutaneous spider angiomata, Dupuytren's contractures). Acanthosis nigricans may reflect underlying cancer (especially gastric cancer). Cutaneous telangiectases of skin or mucous membranes and lips raise the possibility of hereditary hemorrhagic telangiectasia (Osler-Weber-Rendu disease); pigmented lip lesions are seen with Peutz-Jeghers syndrome; cutaneous tumors suggest neurofibromatosis; and purpura is consistent with vascular disease (Henoch-Schönlein purpura or polyarteritis nodosa). Abdominal tenderness (peptic ulcer, pancreatitis, and ischemia), abdominal masses, lymphadenopathy (malignancy), and splenomegaly (cirrhosis, splenic vein thrombosis) are all important to detect.

Hematemesis, melena, and hematochezia are classic symptoms and signs of gastrointestinal bleeding. It requires at least 50 mL of blood in the upper gastrointestinal tract for melena to become clinically apparent, although volumes of up to 100 mL of blood when infused into the stomach may be clinically silent [7]. When bright red blood is vomited, this typically signifies upper gastrointestinal bleeding that is significant, and is often caused by varices or an arterial lesion. Smaller amounts of bleeding from many other lesions are alarming to patients, however, and are often reported. Careful inquiry about the volume of vomited blood is essential. Witness of the amount of and character of blood may also be useful in ascertaining the character of bleeding. Patients with coffee ground emesis are not usually bleeding actively but have had a recent or even remote bleed. Although hematochezia can be caused by bleeding from many different sites in the gastrointestinal tract, the higher the site of bleeding the more hemodynamically significant. Small amounts of hematochezia are often reported by the patient, and care should be taken to ascertain the volume of blood. Chronic occult blood loss may lead to end-organ symptoms, such as lightheadedness, dyspnea, angina pectoris, or even myocardial infarction.

Bedside examination of the character of the stool is an essential and mandatory part of the physical examination. This part of the examination provides critical information about the site of bleeding, and also about the acuity of bleeding. For example, patients who are passing stools containing red blood, maroon-colored blood, or melena have active bleeding. In contrast, patients with brown stools are unlikely to have aggressive bleeding. Likewise, patients with infrequent stools are unlikely to have active bleeding, and those with a history of coffee ground emesis only and normal-appearing stools, whether positive for occult blood or not, have usually had a trivial bleed.

LABORATORY EVALUATION

Unfortunately, far too great a focus has been historically placed on the hematocrit value in patients with gastrointestinal bleeding. This is because the hematocrit, when determined soon after the onset of bleeding, may not reflect blood loss accurately. For example, the hematocrit during exsanguination may not be substantially depressed until extravascular fluid and subsequent hemodilution take place. A single hematocrit level may not reflect the degree of bleeding. The hematocrit value only falls as extravascular fluid enters the vascular space to restore volume, a process that is typically complete after 24 to 72 hours [8].

Another situation that must be recognized in patients with gastrointestinal bleeding is in the subset of patients who bleed small amounts of blood over long periods of time and develop iron deficiency. Although these patients typically have low hematocrits (and indeed they may be very low), they are often hemodynamically stable. A low mean corpuscular volume is often an important clue in these patients, and complemented by a low ferritin level, makes the diagnosis of iron deficiency. This clinical scenario emphasizes that the hematocrit must always be judged in the context of the patient's overall clinical state.

The blood urea nitrogen level may be elevated in patients with upper gastrointestinal bleeding. The elevation is typically out of proportion to elevation in the serum creatinine level [9] because of breakdown of blood proteins to urea by intestinal bacteria and its absorption, and from a mild reduction in the glomerular filtration rate.

CLINICAL LOCALIZATION OF BLEEDING

The localization of bleeding should begin with the history and physical examination and should be focused immediately, during hemodynamic stabilization. Hematemesis denotes an upper gastrointestinal source of bleeding. Melena indicates that blood has been in the gastrointestinal tract for extended periods of time and is usually the result of upper gastrointestinal bleeding, but its source may be the distal small bowel or even the ascending colon. In the latter instance, the volume of bleeding is too little to cause hematochezia but sufficiently large to provide hemoglobin for degradation. Approximately 10% of all patients with rapid bleeding from an upper source present with hematochezia [10]. In these patients, bleeding is typically brisk.

The nasogastric lavage has been commonly used to help differentiate upper from lower gastrointestinal bleeding [11,12]. A bloody aspirate indicates that the upper gastrointestinal tract is the source of bleeding, because the false-positive rate is extremely low, and is usually caused by nasogastric trauma [12]. The nasogastric lavage is frequently used to judge the acuity of bleeding. This approach, however, may be problematic because it may be extremely difficult to judge the acuity or activity of bleeding and the physician assessment of bleeding is weak, with 79% sensitivity and 55% specificity for active bleeding [11]. Primary use of the nasogastric lavage to assess bleeding activity is discouraged. Assessment of vital signs and the use of bedside diagnostic criteria as previously mentioned is a more effective means to determine the activity of bleeding. Further, a positive nasogastric lavage does not provide information about the etiology of bleeding.

Although a nonbloody nasogastric aspirate suggests that bleeding is from a source other than the upper gastrointestinal tract, it is negative in up to 25% of patients with upper gastrointestinal bleeding. Even a bile-colored aspirate, which signifies sampling of the duodenum, does not exclude an upper gastrointestinal source of bleeding. If there is any question about the location of bleeding in a patient with hematochezia, especially in patients with hemodynamic instability, a nasogastric tube should be placed. Testing for occult blood in nasogastric aspirates, although commonly performed, is rarely necessary and helpful only when a coffee ground appearance of the aspirate may be caused by some foods. Although nasogastric tubes are useful to help determine the site of bleeding and to help direct further investigation, there is no evidence that their use affects the outcome.

Other clues that can help localize an upper gastrointestinal source of bleeding include hyperactive bowel sounds and an elevation in the blood urea nitrogen level out of proportion to creatinine. For example, in a series of patients with gastrointestinal bleeding, the mean ($\pm$ SD) blood urea nitrogen/creatinine ratio was significantly higher in patients with upper gastrointestinal bleeding than in those with lower gastrointestinal bleeding (22.5 $\pm$ 11.5 versus 15.9 $\pm$ 8.2; $P = .0001$) [9]. The degree of overlap, however, indicates that the blood urea nitrogen/creatinine ratio has poor discriminatory value.

DIAGNOSIS AND THERAPY

Diagnostic tests play a central role in the evaluation of patients with gastrointestinal bleeding. The major categories of tests available include the following: (1) endoscopy; (2) barium radiographs; (3) radionuclide imaging; (4) angiography; and (5) miscellaneous tests (ie, abdominal CT scanning). The radiographic tests allow diagnosis only, whereas endoscopic tests allow both diagnosis and therapy. The importance of endoscopic therapy is emphasized by studies performed before the advent of endoscopic therapy, which demonstrated that endoscopy per se did not affect outcome for patients with upper gastrointestinal bleeding [13].

A major goal of treatment is to stop active bleeding and prevent recurrent bleeding. The major forms of therapy include (1) pharmacologic, (2) endoscopic, (3) angiographic, and (4) surgical. The use of each of these modalities has undergone tremendous change over the past two decades. Importantly, the use of each diagnostic test and therapeutic intervention varies with the cause of bleeding. They are each often complementary and require focused, multispecialty expertise. Detailed approaches are highlighted elsewhere in this issue in articles that deal with specific types of gastrointestinal bleeding.

References

[1] Rubin TA, Murdoch M, Nelson DB. Acute GI bleeding in the setting of supratherapeutic international normalized ratio in patients taking warfarin: endoscopic diagnosis, clinical management, and outcomes. Gastrointest Endosc 2003;58:369.

[2] Schiff L, Stevens RJ, Shapiro N, et al. Observations on the oral administration of citrate blood in man. Am J Med Sci 1942;203:409.

[3] Ebert RA, Stead EA, Gibson JG. Response of normal subjects to acute blood loss. Arch Intern Med 1940;68:578.

[4] Gilbert DA. Epidemiology of upper gastrointestinal bleeding. Gastrointest Endosc 1990;36:S8.

[5] Cuellar RE, Gavaler JS, Alexander JA, et al. Gastrointestinal tract hemorrhage: the value of a nasogastric aspirate [see comments]. Arch Intern Med 1990;150:1381.

[6] Peterson WL, Barnett CC, Smith HJ, et al. Routine early endoscopy in upper-gastrointestinal-tract bleeding: a randomized, controlled trial. N Engl J Med 1981;304:925.

[7] Luk GD, Bynum TE, Hendrix TR. Gastric aspiration in localization of gastrointestinal hemorrhage. JAMA 1979;241:576.

[8] Baradarian R, Ramdhaney S, Chapalamadugu R, et al. Early intensive resuscitation of patients with upper gastrointestinal bleeding decreases mortality. Am J Gastroenterol 2004;99:619.

[9] Longstreth GF. Epidemiology and outcome of patients hospitalized with acute lower gastro-intestinal hemorrhage: a population-based study. Am J Gastroenterol 1997;92:419.

[10] Segal WN, Cello JP. Hemorrhage in the upper gastrointestinal tract in the older patient. Am J Gastroenterol 1997;92:42.

[11] Longstreth GF. Epidemiology of hospitalization for acute upper gastrointestinal hemor-rhage: a population-based study [see comments]. Am J Gastroenterol 1995;90:206.

[12] Chalasani N, Clark WS, Wilcox CM. Blood urea nitrogen to creatinine concentration in gastrointestinal bleeding: a reappraisal [see comments]. Am J Gastroenterol 1997;92:1796.

[13] Jensen DM, Machicado GA. Diagnosis and treatment of severe hematochezia: the role of urgent colonoscopy after purge. Gastroenterology 1988;95:1569.

GASTROENTEROLOGY CLINICS
OF NORTH AMERICA

ELSEVIER
SAUNDERS

Nonvariceal Upper Gastrointestinal Bleeding: Epidemiology and Diagnosis

Eric Esrailian, MD, Ian M. Gralnek, MD, MSHS*

David Geffen School of Medicine at UCLA, VA Greater Los Angeles Healthcare System,
UCLA/VA Center for Outcomes Research and Education, 11301 Wilshire Boulevard,
CURE Building 115, Room 215, Los Angeles, CA 90073, USA

Despite recent advances in both gastrointestinal endoscopy and the understanding of the pathophysiology of peptic ulcer disease, upper gastrointestinal bleeding (UGIB) remains a significant cause of both morbidity and mortality. Traditionally, UGIB is categorized as being either variceal or nonvariceal, and this article focuses exclusively on the epidemiology and diagnosis of nonvariceal UGIB. Variceal bleeding and the various approaches to its diagnosis and management are addressed elsewhere in this issue.

EPIDEMIOLOGY
Incidence and Demographics

Acute UGIB remains a common medical problem that has significant associated morbidity, mortality, and health care resource use [1]. Early studies performed in the 1970s and 1980s to estimate the magnitude of clinical burden associated with UGIB were limited by their sample size or flaws in methodology. Single-center studies and case series were important initially, but large population-based studies and collaborative databases are now contributing to the increasing knowledge on acute, nonvariceal UGIB. In the past decade, the body of literature on this topic has steadily grown. Based on two large studies from the United Kingdom, the estimated annual incidence of acute UGIB is approximated between 103 and 172 per 100,000 population [2,3]. Incidence rates cited in studies vary given differences in sample populations and study methods. For example, the aforementioned incidence rates are more than twice the rates reported (45–47.7 per 100,000 population) in similar studies from The Netherlands [4,5]. A recent analysis of the Canadian Registry on Nonvariceal Upper Gastrointestinal Bleeding and Endoscopy database of 1869 patients revealed a mean age of 66 years and a predominance of males among patients with nonvariceal UGIB [6]. These findings are summarized in Table 1 [6].

*Corresponding author. E-mail address: i_gralnek@rambam.health.gov.il (I.M. Gralnek).

0889-8553/05/$ – see front matter
doi:10.1016/j.gtc.2005.08.006

Table 1
Canadian Registry on Nonvariceal Upper Gastrointestinal Bleeding and Endoscopy findings for 1869 patients

Finding	Mean value (%)	SD/Cl$_{95}$
Male	62	59.7–64.1
Age (y)	66	+/−17
Past history of UGIB	19.5	17.1–20.9
Past history of PUD	27	23.9–28.1
Number of comorbidities	2.5	+/−1.6
Presenting sign		
Melena	69	67.2–71.4
Hematemesis	30	27.5–31.6
Coffee-ground emesis	28	25.8–29.8
Hematochezia	15	13.6–16.9
Rectal examination yield		
Melena	25	22.7–26.6
Bright red blood	5	4.3–6.4
OB+ stool	25	23.1–27.1
NGT findings		
Coffee-ground material	11	9.9–12.8
Bright red blood	9	7.4–9.9

Abbreviations: Cl$_{95}$, 95% confidence interval; NGT, nasogastric tube aspiration; OB+, occult blood positive; PUD, pepticulcer disease; SD, standard deviation; UGIB, upper gastrointestinal bleeding.

Adapted from Barkun A, Sabbah S, Enns R, et al. The Canadian Registry on Nonvariceal Upper Gastrointestinal Bleeding and Endoscopy (RUGBE): endoscopic hemostasis and proton pump inhibition are associated with improved outcomes in a real-life setting. Am J Gastroenterol 2004;99:1238–46; with permission.

Several population-based and prospective studies support peptic ulcer disease (PUD) being the most common cause of acute UGIB (Fig. 1) [7]. PUD traditionally refers to either gastric or duodenal ulcers, but under a broad heading of "ulcers" some investigators also include esophageal ulcers [6]. Approximately 50% of all cases of acute UGIB are attributed to PUD, and it has long been suggested to be the most common cause of nonvariceal UGIB [8–10]. Recent evidence suggests, however, that the incidence of PUD as a cause of acute UGIB may either be decreasing or is underreported. For example, in an analysis of the Clinical Outcomes Research Initiative (CORI) database between December 1999 and July 2001 (Fig. 2), endoscopy performed for acute UGIB found a duodenal or gastric ulcer in only 1610 (20.6%) of 7822 patients [11]. This study reported "mucosal abnormality" as being the most common endoscopic finding (40%) in persons with acute UGIB. CORI is a consortium of practice sites that use a structured endoscopy reporting system to collect information in a national endoscopic database. CORI currently receives more than 220,000 endoscopic reports annually from 73 practice sites in 24 states [12]. The CORI data are useful because they reflect endoscopic practice from a wide-range of practice settings and minimize patient selection bias. Widespread proton pump inhibitor prescribing and *Helicobacter pylori* eradication

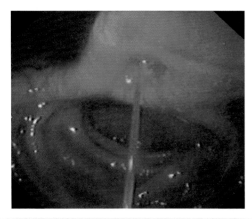

Fig. 1. Spurting gastric ulcer. (Courtesy of UCLA CURE Hemostasis Group, with permission.)

protocols also likely contribute to this observed downward incidence trend of PUD causing nonvariceal UGIB.

Another recently reported trend in acute UGIB involves cyclooxygenase-2 inhibitors. Cyclooxygenase-2 inhibitors are extensively used for both their anti-inflammatory and analgesic properties and their potential for decreased gastrointestinal toxicity. This class of anti-inflammatory drugs is associated with both decreased endoscopic lesions and episodes of UGIB when compared with their nonselective nonsteroidal anti-inflammatory drug counterparts [13–16]. Evidence suggests that the introduction of cyclooxygenase-2 inhibitors may be associated with an overall increased nonsteroidal anti-inflammatory

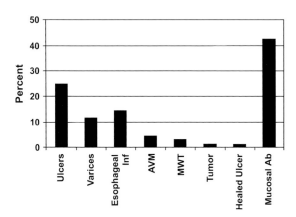

Fig. 2. Endoscopic findings for UGIB from the CORI database. AVM, arteriovenous malformation; Esophageal Inf, esophageal inflammation; Mucosal AB, mucosal abnormality; MWT, Mallory-Weiss tear. (*Adapted from* Boonpongmanee S, Fleischer DE, Pezzullo JC, et al. The frequency of peptic ulcer as a cause of upper-GI bleeding is exaggerated. Gastrointest Endosc 2004;59:788–94; with permission.)

drug use and UGIB on a population-based level [17]. Independently, odds ratios in studies also suggest a relationship between cyclooxygenase-2 inhibitors and UGIB [18]. Gastrointestinal hemorrhage can certainly be facilitated when a patient has an endogenous coagulopathic state or is taking anticoagulation therapy. Nonselective nonsteroidal anti-inflammatory drugs and cyclooxygenase-2 inhibitors both seem to be associated with an increased risk of UGIB when taken concomitantly with warfarin [19].

Classically, Mallory-Weiss tears are mucosal lacerations at the gastroesophageal junction or in the cardia of the stomach [20]. These lesions can be associated with repeated retching or vomiting and are another important cause of nonvariceal UGIB. It is estimated that 5% to 15% of all cases of acute UGIB are secondary to Mallory-Weiss tears [21–23]. Most bleeding episodes caused by Mallory-Weiss tears are self-limited and do not require endoscopic hemostasis [24]. Nevertheless, some cases are severe enough to require blood transfusions, endoscopic hemostasis, interventional radiology, or surgery.

Vascular ectasias, also referred to as "angiomas," "arteriovenous malformations," and "angiodysplasia," are another source of acute and chronic nonvariceal UGIB [25]. Vascular ectasias are the underlying etiology of acute UGIB in approximately 5% to 10% of cases and the severity of bleeding can also range from trivial to severe. Vascular ectasias are associated with chronic renal insufficiency or failure [26–29]; valvular heart disease, specifically aortic stenosis; and congestive heart failure [30,31]. The evidence for these associations is limited, however, and association does not equal causation [32]. It is more likely that UGIB from pre-existing vascular ectasias is facilitated by acquired von Willebrand's disease [33,34].

Isolated vascular ectasias are endoscopically different than the diffuse linear array seen in gastric antral vascular ectasia, also referred to as "watermelon stomach" [35,36]. Gastric antral vascular ectasia is thought to be a distinct clinical entity from portal hypertensive gastropathy and is characterized by red stripes interposed by normal-appearing mucosa generally noted in the gastric antrum, yet lesions in the proximal stomach and cardia may also be observed [37]. Unlike portal hypertensive gastropathy, many patients with gastric antral vascular ectasia do not have portal hypertension [38] and the etiology of gastric antral vascular ectasia and its differences from portal hypertensive gastropathy have yet to be fully explained [39].

Dieulafoy's lesion is a rare etiology in acute UGIB (Fig. 3). These were first described by Gallard [40] in 1884, and subsequently Dieulafoy [41] in 1898. Dieulafoy's lesions are difficult to identify endoscopically because they often retract. Their histopathologic description is a "caliber-persistent artery" in the submucosal tissue [42]. These lesions represent the etiology for nonvariceal UGIB in less than 5% of all UGIB cases [43,44]. On endoscopy, a Dieulafoy's lesion is akin to a visible vessel protruding from an ulcer, yet without an underlying ulcer. A formal assessment of endoscopic criteria does allow for a minute mucosal defect to be present, but such definitions are subjective and likely impact prevalence of these lesions [45].

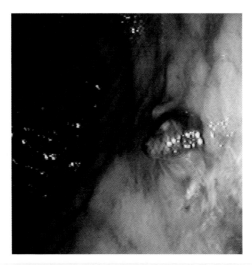

Fig. 3. Dieulafoy's lesion in the stomach. (Courtesy of UCLA CURE Hemostasis Group, with permission.)

Neoplasms, both malignant and benign, are another infrequent cause of nonvariceal UGIB and comprise less than 5% of all UGIB cases [46]. Although neoplasms make up a small fraction of overall bleeding episodes, UGIB can be a common presenting sign for a neoplasm and should be part of the differential diagnosis [47]. The lesion can be a primary malignancy, such as esophageal, gastric, or duodenal adenocarcinoma; esophageal squamous cell carcinoma; gastric or duodenal lymphoma; or a gastrointestinal stromal cell tumor. Metastases, such as those from the colon, lung, and breast, may also be responsible for UGIB [48]. Examples of benign neoplasms that can lead to UGIB include carcinoid tumors, lipomas, and blue rubber bleb nevus syndrome [49–52].

Other rare causes of nonvariceal UGIB should also be considered in any differential diagnosis. For example, aortoenteric fistula must be considered in patients with a history of intra-abdominal vascular surgery, such as an abdominal aortic aneurysm repair [53]. Hemobilia is another rare cause of UGIB that should be considered in the setting of recent hepatobiliary tree instrumentation, such as with endoscopic retrograde cholangiopancreatography or laparoscopic cholecystectomy. Bile duct and hepatic artery injuries are possible complications of these procedures, and patients can ultimately present with signs of UGIB [54]. In patients with chronic pancreatitis who present with acute UGIB, hemosuccus pancreaticus should also be excluded. Although it is an uncommon cause of UGIB overall, bleeding in these patients can be secondary to a pseudoaneurysm in peripancreatic blood vessels as a complication of pancreatic pseudocysts [55]. Finally, iatrogenic injuries secondary to endoscopic procedures, such as percutaneous endoscopic gastrostomy tube placement, are also rare causes of nonvariceal UGIB [56].

Mortality rates associated with acute, nonvariceal UGIB also vary depending on the study and the risk for an individual patient depends on specific factors, such as the severity of the bleeding episode, comorbidities, and the underlying bleeding etiology. Mortality as high as 36% in cases of nonvariceal UGIB has been reported [57]. Most studies document mortality rates of approximately 10%, however, and these figures have not dramatically changed over the past two decades [58–60]. The evolution of acid-suppression therapy (eg, proton pump inhibitors) has been an important development over the past 20 years. Although these pharmacologic agents have improved rebleeding rates and decreased the need for surgery, mortality has not been significantly affected [61]. An aging population with increased comorbidities may be one contributing factor. A recent study of nearly 2000 Canadian patients documented a mortality rate of 5.4% [6]. Resuscitation is discussed in the article addressing management and therapy of nonvariceal UGIB elsewhere in this issue. Aggressive resuscitation may have the potential to improve mortality [62].

Nonvariceal UGIB results in a tremendous use of health care resources and consequently an economic burden [63]. Direct costs include ICU stays, hospital bed-days, gastrointestinal endoscopy, laboratory tests, and blood product transfusions. Data on exact cost figures from acute UGIB are limited but are estimated to be several thousand dollars per bleeding episode with annual direct cost projections being estimated at approximately $1 billion dollars [64–67].

In the discipline of health services, a framework of health care quality consists of three components: (1) structure, (2) process, and (3) outcome [68]. Process of care refers to the details of the provider-patient interaction. Variation in process of care for nonvariceal UGIB may be an important factor contributing to observed large variations in the costs associated with bleeding episodes. Evidence suggests that disparities in the practice patterns of different specialties may be one reason for this variation [69,70]. Patterns of care across alternative medical settings may also contribute to this variation. For example, a study comparing tertiary medical centers in the United States and Canada documented variation in the process of care for persons presenting with acute nonvariceal UGIB. This study, however, did not demonstrate significant differences in clinical outcome. In light of these findings, care pathways have been developed to limit this variation and control costs. Specific management strategies for persons with acute UGIB are addressed elsewhere in this issue [71].

DIAGNOSIS

Clinical Presentation and Patient Triage

A thorough medical history and careful physical examination are critical in the assessment of an individual presenting with gastrointestinal bleeding. Details from the patient history can help mold the differential diagnosis and stratify patient outcomes. A history of taking nonsteroidal anti-inflammatory drugs, aspirin, antiplatelet agents, or anticoagulation therapies, such as warfarin, are important pieces of information to acquire during the history. A history of documented PUD with previous UGIB, known *H pylori* infection, and compliance with proton pump inhibitor therapy are also important issues to address. Furthermore, the aforementioned relationship between advanced age, chronic renal insufficiency, valvular heart disease, and vascular ectasias should be noted. Advanced patient age also increases the likelihood of a gastrointestinal neoplasm as a possible etiology [12,72]. Finally, known history of liver disease risk factors should make the clinician aware of the possibility of esophagogastric variceal hemorrhage.

The physical examination should be focused, yet complete. Vital signs should be obtained including evaluation for evidence of orthostasis. The presence or absence of orthostatic hypotension provides an indication of the patient's volume status and can help guide volume resuscitation. Mucous membranes and neck veins should also be evaluated as additional ways of estimating patient volume status. In addition, the examiner should look carefully for scleral icterus, conjunctival pallor, and telangiectasias on the lips or oropharynx. The abdominal examination should include visual observation for distention; auscultation for presence of bowel sounds (or lack thereof, which may be seen in viscus perforation); and palpation for tenderness, organomegaly, guarding, rebound, and shifting dullness. The skin examination should include observation for jaundice, tenting, spider angiomas, and palmar erythema.

Hematemesis and melena are important clinical signs highly suggestive of an upper gastrointestinal tract (proximal to the ligament of Treitz) source of hemorrhage. Less frequently, patients with distal small bowel bleeding or a right-sided colonic lesion in the setting of slow colonic transit time may also present with melena. Similarly, a presentation with hematochezia does not solely indicate bleeding from the distal small bowel or colon [73]. Subjective reporting of stool color by patients is fallible and should not preclude a systematic evaluation for a source of gastrointestinal hemorrhage [74]. Personal evaluation by the clinician by digital rectal examination is a key component of the physical examination in all cases of gastrointestinal bleeding. Patients with UGIB can present with hematochezia, yet this scenario is less common. UGIB presenting with hematochezia is indicative of brisk bleeding and is often seen in concert with hemodynamic instability, but the possibility of UGIB should still be kept in the differential diagnosis even in patients who initially seem to be hemodynamically stable [75]. Moreover, severe UGIB may be painless, and the absence of pain should not preclude an appropriate evaluation for an upper gastrointestinal source of hemorrhage [76].

Certain laboratory tests are useful during initial assessment of the patient. Hemoglobin and hematocrit levels, and the subsequent response to transfusions if needed, is part of the decision-making process when diagnosing UGIB. The initial hemoglobin value, and especially the hematocrit, may not reflect a patient's true blood level and may be falsely elevated because of hemoconcentration. In patients with recent bleeding, it may take several hours for the equilibration of hemoglobin concentration to be reflected accurately on a complete blood count. In the setting of active bleeding, the values in the complete blood count are likely to be dynamic even with vigorous resuscitation efforts. If a patient seems to be euvolemic and has not recently bled, however, the hemoglobin and hematocrit may equilibrate rapidly after blood transfusion [77,78].

In addition to the complete blood count, other laboratory values can be complementary to the history and physical examination in the diagnosis of acute UGIB and include platelet count; prothrombin time and international normalized ratio; and if suspected underlying liver disease, liver tests. Because of an increased protein load from digested blood in the proximal gastrointestinal tract, an elevated serum blood urea nitrogen out of proportion to an increase in serum creatinine may be suggestive of UGIB [79,80]. Although an elevated blood urea nitrogen to creatinine ratio may be indicative of UGIB, this ratio is not specific and can also represent intravascular volume depletion and a resultant prerenal azotemia [81]. Leukocytosis can also be seen on the complete blood count in acute UGIB. Physiologic stress-induced demargination of leukocytes can be responsible for this finding and does not necessarily indicate an underlying infectious process [82]. The white blood cell differential should also be noted to assess for neutrophilia and bandemia, which can be more suggestive of an infection. Nevertheless, if clinical suspicion of infection warrants further investigation, then appropriate cultures should be collected in patients with leukocytosis and UGIB.

Nasogastric tube aspiration can be an important component of the evaluation of UGIB. Studies evaluating the usefulness of nasogastric tube aspiration in predicting high-risk lesions, such as a peptic ulcer with active bleeding or a visible vessel, have produced large variations in sensitivity, specificity, and positive and negative predictive values [83]. Interpretation of the nasogastric tube aspirate by the clinician at the point of contact, usually in the emergency department, is subjective and often reported to a consulting gastroenterologist secondhand. In general, overtly bloody nasogastric tube aspirates are correlated with high-risk endoscopic lesions in the upper gastrointestinal tract [84–86]. Clinicians often question the need for an nasogastric tube in the setting of melena or hematemesis. Nasogastric tube placement does not serve a purely diagnostic purpose, however, and can be useful for gastric lavage and has the potential to minimize the aspiration risk from a blood-filled stomach in preparation for endoscopy [87]. Specifically, gastric lavage has been shown to improve visualization of the gastric fundus when performed before endoscopy for acute UGIB [88]. Other authorities question this practice because of the potential for aspiration and suggest a large-bore orogastric tube inserted through an overtube [89].

To risk stratify individuals presenting with acute UGIB better, risk scoring tools have been developed to facilitate patient triage, predict risk of rebleeding and mortality, evaluate need for ICU admission, and determine need for urgent endoscopy [90]. These scoring tools have been almost exclusively used in research studies, and are uncommonly applied in everyday clinical practice [91]. Some risk scoring tools, such as the Blatchford Score, use laboratory findings, patient vital signs at presentation, and other clinical variables without the use of endoscopy [92]. A major limitation for interpreting the results of studies evaluating risk scoring tools that do not use endoscopic findings is the lack of large, prospective trials [93]. A recent study compared risk-scoring tools that use clinical and endoscopic variables with those that use only clinical variables to quantify the incremental value of endoscopy in the identification of patients at low-risk for recurrent bleeding and mortality. The complete Rockall Score identified significantly more low-risk patients with acute UGIB than either the clinical Rockall Score or the Blatchford Score [94]. Risk stratification may be important because of the potential to minimize the unnecessary use of hospital-based services, iatrogenic complications, and worker absenteeism. Artificial neural networks use computer science principles to simulate biologic processes. Artificial neural networks have also been used for risk stratification and to predict outcome in lower gastrointestinal bleeding [95]. Artificial neural networks and other risk stratification devices that do not use endoscopic findings may be useful when endoscopy is not available. Nevertheless, clinicians should continue to use evidence-based approaches and remain aware that medical decision-making can be dynamic and exceptions may exist for various treatment algorithms [96].

Gastrointestinal Endoscopy

Endoscopy is the best tool for both the diagnosis and ultimately as a therapeutic measure for patients with acute UGIB. Improvements in endoscopic technology and operator skill have clearly reduced the need for surgery and interventional radiology as diagnostic and therapeutic procedures for UGIB. Patient positioning before and during the procedure can assist with improving visibility during endoscopy [89]. Positioning the patient with the bleeding point in the most superior position can help clear the endoscopic field by allowing blood to flow away from the point of bleeding. Reverse Trendelenburg positioning and rolling the patient from the left lateral decubitus position to the right and back can also be used to move clots and blood away from dependent areas in the stomach. The choice of endoscope is also a critical aspect of making an accurate diagnosis for nonvariceal UGIB. A large single-channel or double-channel therapeutic endoscope should be used in all cases of suspected acute UGIB. This technique should be used both for the ability to suction larger volumes of gastroduodenal contents and for the potential to provide hemostasis therapy using a large-size (10F catheter) thermal probe or mechanical clipping device.

Early endoscopy, generally defined as within 24 hours of patient hospital presentation or admission, has been shown to reduce resource use, decrease transfusion requirements, and shorten hospital stay [97,98]. There is conflicting evidence whether or not performing endoscopy even earlier (eg, in the emergency department) can further decrease resource use and minimize health care costs. Lee and colleagues [99] demonstrated a significant decrease in hospital costs and duration of stay with endoscopic triage performed in the emergency department. Conversely, Bjorkman and colleagues [100] found that urgent endoscopy failed to decrease health care resource use. These authors cited a disconnect between consulting endoscopists and admitting primary care or emergency department physicians as a key factor for their findings.

Endoscopy should be the primary procedure performed for the diagnosis of UGIB once standard pre-endoscopy criteria are met [101]. Although some analyses reveal endoscopy may be inappropriately overused, the technique has a high yield in making the diagnosis of UGIB, and the procedure is clearly indicated in this setting [102,103]. In general, gastrointestinal endoscopy is considered safe and well-tolerated even among elderly patients [104]. The presence of blood in the stomach on upper endoscopy is an important finding when assessing risk initially [105]. For PUD, risk-stratification and evidence-based prediction of rebleeding potential is possible using endoscopic findings. Table 2 details the prevalence and outcomes of PUD using endoscopic stigmata. Active bleeding (spurting or oozing) or a nonbleeding visible vessel seen on endoscopy have the highest potential for rebleeding with rates of approximately 55% and 43%, respectively (see Fig. 3). This knowledge can guide the decision for discharge, hospital admission, or admission to an ICU. Despite the importance of making an accurate diagnosis, evidence suggests that there is frequent intraobserver variability on grading endoscopic stigmata [106,107].

If there is clinical evidence of recurrent bleeding after primary hemostasis has been achieved, esophagogastroduodenoscopy should be repeated with a view toward repeat hemostasis if needed [108]. In UGIB secondary to PUD, rebleeding occurs in approximately 10% to 30% of patients who have high-risk stigmata (active bleeding, nonbleeding visible vessel, adherent clot) at the time of initial esophagogastroduodenoscopy and who receive endoscopic hemostasis [109]. In addition, evidence from recent studies suggests that performing a second-look endoscopy (regardless of any clinical evidence of recurrent hemorrhage) in patients with high-risk ulcer stigmata at the time of their initial esophagogastroduodenoscopy may decrease rebleeding rates, need for surgery, and health care costs [110,111]. The feasibility and importance of

Table 2
Prevalence and outcomes of peptic ulcer disease based on endoscopic stigmata

Endoscopic characteristics	Forrest classification	Prevalence % (range)	Rebleeding % (range)	Surgery % (range)	Mortality % (range)
Clean base	III	42 (19–52)	5 (0–10)	0.5 (0–3)	2 (0–3)
Pigmented flat spot	IIC	20 (0–42)	10 (0–13)	6 (0–10)	3 (0–10)
Adherent clot	IIB	17 (0–49)	22 (14–36)	10 (5–12)	7 (0–10)
NBVV	IIA	17 (4–35)	43 (0–81)	34 (0–56)	11 (0–21)
Active bleed	IA	18 (4–26)	55 (17–100)	35 (20–69)	11 (0–23)

Abbreviation: NBVV, nonbleeding visible vessel.
   Adapted from Laine L, Peterson WL. Bleeding peptic ulcer. N Engl J Med 1994;331:717–27; with permission.

this in actual clinical practice, however, may be dependent on the health care setting of the patient and provider.

Using ultrasound as an accessory modality for cases of UGIB is not a new concept [112]. Much of the literature surrounding the use of endoscopic ultrasound for UGIB involves gastroesophageal varices and other clinical issues related to portal hypertension [113–115]. The literature on endoscopic ultrasound in nonvariceal UGIB is growing, however, and reports exist of this technique being used as an adjunctive diagnostic tool in a variety of settings including peptic ulcer hemorrhage, Dieulafoy's lesion, and evaluating hemobilia [116,117]. A Doppler ultrasound probe can be passed through the accessory channel of a therapeutic endoscope. A persistent Doppler ultrasound signal after endoscopic hemostasis in PUD has been associated with a higher rebleeding rate, and some authors endorse evaluating for the presence of a Doppler signal before and after hemostasis therapy in PUD so as to ensure better complete hemostasis [118].

Additional Modalities

Angiography and technetium scanning are useful alternatives when endoscopy has not yielded a definitive diagnosis or is unable to be performed. The details of these modalities in the diagnosis and management of gastrointestinal bleeding are discussed elsewhere in this issue. Other radiographic studies may also be useful when making the diagnosis of UGIB, but not usually in the acute setting. An esophagram, or upper gastrointestinal series, and small bowel follow-through were used more for the diagnosis of UGIB before the advances in endoscopic technologies over the past two decades and generally are no longer used as part of the diagnostic evaluation of persons with acute UGIB [119–121].

Wireless capsule endoscopy is now being used as a diagnostic tool for a variety of gastrointestinal disorders including Crohn's disease, celiac disease, and obscure gastrointestinal bleeding [122,123]. At the present time, however, it is not a practical modality to use in acute UGIB. Its clinical use in the evaluation of obscure bleeding is discussed elsewhere in this issue.

References

[1] Dulai GS, Gralnek IM, Oei TT, et al. Utilization of health care resources for low-risk patients with acute, nonvariceal upper GI hemorrhage: an historical cohort study. Gastrointest Endosc 2002;55:321–7.
[2] Rockall TA, Logan RF, Devlin HB, et al. Incidence of and mortality from acute upper gastrointestinal haemorrhage in the United Kingdom. Steering Committee and members of the National Audit of Acute Upper Gastrointestinal Haemorrhage. BMJ 1995;311:222–6.
[3] Blatchford O, Davidson LA, Murray WR, et al. Acute upper gastrointestinal haemorrhage in west of Scotland: case ascertainment study. BMJ 1997;315:510–4.
[4] Vreeburg EM, Snel P, de Bruijne JW, et al. Acute upper gastrointestinal bleeding in the Amsterdam area: incidence, diagnosis, and clinical outcome. Am J Gastroenterol 1997;92:236–43.
[5] van Leerdam ME, Vreeburg EM, Rauws EA, et al. Acute upper GI bleeding: did anything change? Time trend analysis of incidence and outcome of acute upper GI bleeding between 1993/1994 and 2000. Am J Gastroenterol 2003;98:1494–9.

[6] Barkun A, Sabbah S, Enns R, et al. The Canadian Registry on Nonvariceal Upper Gastro-intestinal Bleeding and Endoscopy (RUGBE): endoscopic hemostasis and proton pump inhibition are associated with improved outcomes in a real-life setting. Am J Gastroenterol 2004;99:1238–46.

[7] Jensen DM. Endoscopic control of non-variceal upper gastrointestinal hemorrhage. In: Yamada T, Alpers D, Laine L, et al, editors. Textbook of gastroenterology. 3rd edition. Philadelphia: Lippincott; 1999. p. 2857–79.

[8] Silverstein FE, Gilbert DA, Tedesco FJ, et al. The national ASGE survey on upper gastro-intestinal bleeding. I. Study design and baseline data. Gastrointest Endosc 1981;27:73–9.

[9] Longstreth GF. Epidemiology of hospitalization for acute upper gastrointestinal hemor-rhage: a population-based study. Am J Gastroenterol 1995;90:206–10.

[10] Peura DA, Lanza FL, Gostout CJ, et al. The American College of Gastroenterology Bleeding Registry: preliminary findings. Am J Gastroenterol 1997;92:924–8.

[11] Boonpongmanee S, Fleischer DE, Pezzullo JC, et al. The frequency of peptic ulcer as a cause of upper-GI bleeding is exaggerated. Gastrointest Endosc 2004;59:788–94.

[12] Lieberman D, Fennerty MB, Morris CD, et al. Endoscopic evaluation of patients with dys-pepsia: results from the national endoscopic data repository. Gastroenterology 2004; 127:1067–75.

[13] Langman MJ, Jensen DM, Watson DJ, et al. Adverse upper gastrointestinal effects of rofe-coxib compared with NSAIDs. JAMA 1999;282:1929–33.

[14] Emery P, Zeidler H, Kvien TK, et al. Celecoxib versus diclofenac in long-term manage-ment of rheumatoid arthritis: randomised double-blind comparison. Lancet 1999;354: 2106–11.

[15] Hunt RH, Harper S, Watson DJ, et al. The gastrointestinal safety of the COX-2 selective in-hibitor etoricoxib assessed by both endoscopy and analysis of upper gastrointestinal events. Am J Gastroenterol 2003;98:1725–33.

[16] Goldstein JL, Eisen GM, Agrawal N, et al. Reduced incidence of upper gastrointestinal ul-cer complications with the COX-2 selective inhibitor, valdecoxib. Aliment Pharmacol Ther 2004;20:527–38.

[17] Mamdani M, Juurlink DN, Kopp A, et al. Gastrointestinal bleeding after the introduction of COX 2 inhibitors: ecological study. BMJ 2004;328:1415–6.

[18] Laporte JR, Ibanez L, Vidal X, et al. Upper gastrointestinal bleeding associated with the use of NSAIDs: newer versus older agents. Drug Saf 2004;27:411–20.

[19] Battistella M, Mamdami MM, Juurlink DN, et al. Risk of upper gastrointestinal hemorrhage in warfarin users treated with nonselective NSAIDs or COX-2 inhibitors. Arch Intern Med 2005;165:189–92.

[20] Mallory GK, Weiss S. Hemorrhages from lacerations of the cardiac orifice of the stomach due to vomiting. Am J Med Sci 1929;178:506–12.

[21] Wilcox CM, Alexander LN, Straub RF, et al. A prospective endoscopic evaluation of the causes of upper GI hemorrhage in alcoholics: a focus on alcoholic gastropathy. Am J Gas-troenterol 1996;91:1343–7.

[22] Llach J, Elizalde JI, Guevara MC, et al. Endoscopic injection therapy in bleeding Mal-lory-Weiss syndrome: a randomized controlled trial. Gastrointest Endosc 2001;54: 679–81.

[23] Huang SP, Wang HP, Lee YC, et al. Endoscopic hemoclip placement and epinephrine in-jection for Mallory-Weiss syndrome with active bleeding. Gastrointest Endosc 2002;55: 842–6.

[24] Morales P, Baum AE. Therapeutic alternatives for the Mallory-Weiss tear. Curr Treat Op-tions Gastroenterol 2003;6:75–83.

[25] Cheng CL, Lee CS, Liu NJ, et al. Overlooked lesions at emergency endoscopy for acute nonvariceal upper gastrointestinal bleeding. Endoscopy 2002;34:527–30.

[26] Zuckerman GR, Cornette GL, Clouse RE, et al. Upper gastrointestinal bleeding in patients with chronic renal failure. Ann Intern Med 1985;102:588–92.

[27] Tsai CJ, Hwang JC. Investigation of upper gastrointestinal hemorrhage in chronic renal failure. J Clin Gastroenterol 1996;22:2–5.
[28] Chalasani N, Cotsonis G, Wilcox CM. Upper gastrointestinal bleeding in patients with chronic renal failure: role of vascular ectasia. Am J Gastroenterol 1996;91:2329–32.
[29] Sotoudehmanesh R, Ali Asgari A, Ansari R, et al. Endoscopic findings in end-stage renal disease. Endoscopy 2003;35:502–5.
[30] Raja K, Kochhar R, Sethy PK, et al. An endoscopic study of upper-GI mucosal changes in patients with congestive heart failure. Gastrointest Endosc 2004;60:887–93.
[31] Batur P, Stewart WJ, Isaacson JH. Increased prevalence of aortic stenosis in patients with arteriovenous malformations of the gastrointestinal tract in Heyde syndrome. Arch Intern Med 2003;163:1821–4.
[32] Bhutani MS, Gupta SC, Markert RJ, et al. A prospective controlled evaluation of endoscopic detection of angiodysplasia and its association with aortic valve disease. Gastrointest Endosc 1995;42:398–402.
[33] Veyradier A, Balian A, Wolf M, et al. Abnormal von Willebrand factor in bleeding angiodysplasias of the digestive tract. Gastroenterology 2001;120:346–53.
[34] Sadler JE. Aortic stenosis, von Willebrand factor, and bleeding. N Engl J Med 2003;349:323–5.
[35] Sebastian S, O'Morain CA, Buckley MJ. Review article: current therapeutic options for gastric antral vascular ectasia. Aliment Pharmacol Ther 2003;18:157–65.
[36] Dulai GS, Jensen DM, Kovacs TO, et al. Endoscopic treatment outcomes in watermelon stomach patients with and without portal hypertension. Endoscopy 2004;36:68–72.
[37] Thuluvath PJ, Yoo HY. Portal hypertensive gastropathy. Am J Gastroenterol 2002;97:2973–8.
[38] Burak KW, Lee SS, Beck PL. Portal hypertensive gastropathy and gastric antral vascular ectasia (GAVE) syndrome. Gut 2001;49:866–72.
[39] Stotzer PO, Willen R, Kilander AF. Watermelon stomach: not only an antral disease. Gastrointest Endosc 2002;55:897–900.
[40] Gallard T. Aneurysmes miliaires de l'estomac donnant lieu à des hématémèses mortelles. [French]. Bull Soc Méd de Hôp Paris 1884;1:84–91.
[41] Dieulafoy G. Exulceratio simplex. Clin méd de l'Hôtel-Dieu de Paris 1897/98, II; L'intervention chirurgicale dans les hématémèses foudroyantes consécutives á l'exulceration simple de l'estomac [French]. Pr Méd 1898;29–44.
[42] Lee YT, Walmsley RS, Leong RW, et al. Dieulafoy's lesion. Gastrointest Endosc 2003;58:236–43.
[43] Romaozinho JM, Pontes JM, Lerias C, et al. Dieulafoy's lesion: management and long-term outcome. Endoscopy 2004;36:416–20.
[44] Park CH, Joo YE, Kim HS, et al. A prospective, randomized trial of endoscopic band ligation versus endoscopic hemoclip placement for bleeding gastric Dieulafoy's lesions. Endoscopy 2004;36:677–81.
[45] Dy NM, Gostout CJ, Balm RK. Bleeding from the endoscopically-identified Dieulafoy lesion of the proximal small intestine and colon. Am J Gastroenterol 1995;90:108–11.
[46] Savides TJ, Jensen DM, Cohen J, et al. Severe upper gastrointestinal tumor bleeding: endoscopic findings, treatment, and outcome. Endoscopy 1996;28:244–8.
[47] Blackshaw GR, Stephens MR, Lewis WG, et al. Prognostic significance of acute presentation with emergency complications of gastric cancer. Gastric Cancer 2004;7:91–6.
[48] Reiman T, Butts CA. Upper gastrointestinal bleeding as a metastatic manifestation of breast cancer: a case report and review of the literature. Can J Gastroenterol 2001;15:67–71.
[49] Roncoroni L, Costi R, Canavese G, et al. Carcinoid tumor associated with vascular malformation as a cause of massive gastric bleeding. Am J Gastroenterol 1997;92:2119–21.
[50] Andersen JM. Blue rubber bleb nevus syndrome. Curr Treat Options Gastroenterol 2001;4:433–40.

[51] Dallal HJ, Ravindran R, King PM, et al. Gastric carcinoid tumour as a cause of severe upper gastrointestinal haemorrhage. Endoscopy 2003;35:716.

[52] Fishman SJ, Smithers CJ, Folkman J, et al. Blue rubber bleb nevus syndrome: surgical eradication of gastrointestinal bleeding. Ann Surg 2005;241:523–8.

[53] Ramanujam S, Shiels A, Zuckerman G, et al. Unusual presentations of aorto-enteric fistula. Gastrointest Endosc 2004;59:300–4.

[54] Chapman WC, Abecassis M, Jarnagin W, et al. Bile duct injuries 12 years after the introduction of laparoscopic cholecystectomy. J Gastrointest Surg 2003;7:412–6.

[55] Elton E, Howell DA, Amberson SM, et al. Combined angiographic and endoscopic management of bleeding pancreatic pseudoaneurysms. Gastrointest Endosc 1997;46: 544–9.

[56] Cappell MS, Abdullah M. Management of gastrointestinal bleeding induced by gastrointestinal endoscopy. Gastroenterol Clin North Am 2000;29:125–67.

[57] Guglielmi A, Ruzzenente A, Sandri M, et al. Risk assessment and prediction of rebleeding in bleeding gastroduodenal ulcer. Endoscopy 2002;34:778–86.

[58] Yavorski RT, Wong RK, Maydonovitch C, et al. Analysis of 3,294 cases of upper gastrointestinal bleeding in military medical facilities. Am J Gastroenterol 1995;90: 568–73.

[59] Rockall TA, Logan RF, Devlin HB, et al. Variation in outcome after acute upper gastrointestinal haemorrhage. The National Audit of Acute Upper Gastrointestinal Haemorrhage. Lancet 1995;346:346–50.

[60] Lewis JD, Bilker WB, Brensinger C, et al. Hospitalization and mortality rates from peptic ulcer disease and GI bleeding in the 1990s: relationship to sales of nonsteroidal anti-inflammatory drugs and acid suppression medications. Am J Gastroenterol 2002;97: 2540–9.

[61] Selby NM, Kubba AK, Hawkey CJ. Acid suppression in peptic ulcer haemorrhage: a meta-analysis. Aliment Pharmacol Ther 2000;14:1119–26.

[62] Baradarian R, Ramdhaney S, Chapalamadugu R, et al. Early intensive resuscitation of patients with upper gastrointestinal bleeding decreases mortality. Am J Gastroenterol 2004;99:619–22.

[63] Lanas A. Economic analysis of strategies in the prevention of non-steroidal anti-inflammatory drug-induced complications in the gastrointestinal tract. Aliment Pharmacol Ther 2004;20:321–31.

[64] Jensen DM. Health and economic aspects of peptic ulcer disease. Am J Med 1984;77: 8–14.

[65] Laine L, Peterson WL. Bleeding peptic ulcer. N Engl J Med 1994;331:717–27.

[66] Gralnek IM, Jensen DM, Kovacs TOG, et al. An economic analysis of patients with active arterial peptic ulcer hemorrhage treated with endoscopic heater probe, injection sclerosis, or surgery in a prospective, randomized trial. Gastrointest Endosc 1997;46:105–12.

[67] Marshall JK, Collins SM, Gafni A. Prediction of resource utilization and case cost for acute nonvariceal upper gastrointestinal hemorrhage at a Canadian community hospital. Am J Gastroenterol 1999;94:1841–6.

[68] Donabedian A. The quality of medical care. Science 1978;200:856–64.

[69] Quirk DM, Barry MJ, Aserkoff B, et al. Physician specialty and variations in the cost of treating patients with acute upper gastrointestinal bleeding. Gastroenterology 1997;113: 1443–8.

[70] Pardo A, Durandez R, Hernandez M, et al. Impact of physician specialty on the cost of nonvariceal upper GI bleeding care. Am J Gastroenterol 2002;97:1535–42.

[71] Pfau PR, Cooper GS, Carlson MD, et al. Success and shortcomings of a clinical care pathway in the management of acute nonvariceal upper gastrointestinal bleeding. Am J Gastroenterol 2004;99:425–31.

[72] Schmidt N, Peitz U, Lippert H, et al. Missing gastric cancer in dyspepsia. Aliment Pharmacol Ther 2005;21:813–20.

[73] Fine KD, Nelson AC, Ellington RT, et al. Comparison of the color of fecal blood with the anatomical location of gastrointestinal bleeding lesions: potential misdiagnosis using only flexible sigmoidoscopy for bright red blood per rectum. Am J Gastroenterol 1999;94:3202–10.

[74] Zuckerman GR, Trellis DR, Sherman TM, et al. An objective measure of stool color for differentiating upper from lower gastrointestinal bleeding. Dig Dis Sci 1995;40:1614–21.

[75] Wilcox CM, Alexander LN, Cotsonis G. A prospective characterization of upper gastrointestinal hemorrhage presenting with hematochezia. Am J Gastroenterol 1997;92:231–5.

[76] Wilcox CM, Clark WS. Features associated with painless peptic ulcer bleeding. Am J Gastroenterol 1997;92:1289–92.

[77] Wiesen AR, Hospenthal DR, Byrd JC, et al. Equilibration of hemoglobin concentration after transfusion in medical inpatients not actively bleeding. Ann Intern Med 1994;121:278–80.

[78] Elizalde JI, Clemente J, Marin JL, et al. Early changes in hemoglobin and hematocrit levels after packed red cell transfusion in patients with acute anemia. Transfusion 1997;37:573–6.

[79] Snook JA, Holdstock GE, Bamforth J. Value of a simple biochemical ratio in distinguishing upper and lower sites of gastrointestinal haemorrhage. Lancet 1986;1:1064–5.

[80] Ernst AA, Haynes ML, Nick TG, et al. Usefulness of the blood urea nitrogen/creatinine ratio in gastrointestinal bleeding. Am J Emerg Med 1999;17:70–2.

[81] Chalasani N, Clark WS, Wilcox CM. Blood urea nitrogen to creatinine concentration in gastrointestinal bleeding: a reappraisal. Am J Gastroenterol 1997;92:1796–9.

[82] Chalasani N, Patel K, Clark WS, et al. The prevalence and significance of leukocytosis in upper gastrointestinal bleeding. Am J Med Sci 1998;315:233–6.

[83] Leung FW. The venerable nasogastric tube. Gastrointest Endosc 2004;59:255–60.

[84] Perng CL, Lin HJ, Chen CJ, et al. Characteristics of patients with bleeding peptic ulcer requiring emergency endoscopy and aggressive treatment. Am J Gastroenterol 1994;89:1811–4.

[85] Peter DJ, Dougherty JM. Evaluation of the patient with gastrointestinal bleeding: an evidence based approach. Emerg Med Clin North Am 1999;17:239–61.

[86] Aljebreen AM, Fallone CA, Barkun AN. Nasogastric aspirate predicts high-risk endoscopic lesions in patients with acute upper-GI bleeding. Gastrointest Endosc 2004;59:172–8.

[87] Stollman NH, Putcha RV, Neustater BR, et al. The uncleared fundal pool in acute upper gastrointestinal bleeding: implications and outcomes. Gastrointest Endosc 1997;46:324–7.

[88] Lee SD, Kearney DJ. A randomized controlled trial of gastric lavage prior to endoscopy for acute upper gastrointestinal bleeding. J Clin Gastroenterol 2004;38:861–5.

[89] Matlock J, Freeman ML. Non-variceal upper GI hemorrhage: doorway to diagnosis. Techniques in Gastrointestinal Endoscopy 2005;7:112–7.

[90] Rockall TA, Logan RF, Devlin HB, et al. Risk assessment after acute upper gastrointestinal haemorrhage. Gut 1996;38:316–21.

[91] Das A, Wong RC. Prediction of outcome of acute GI hemorrhage: a review of risk scores and predictive models. Gastrointest Endosc 2004;60:85–93.

[92] Blatchford O, Murray WR, Blatchford M. A risk score to predict need for treatment for upper-gastrointestinal haemorrhage. Lancet 2000;356:1318–21.

[93] Gralnek IM. Outpatient management of "low-risk" nonvariceal upper GI hemorrhage: are we ready to put evidence into practice? Gastrointest Endosc 2002;55:131–4.

[94] Gralnek IM, Dulai GS. Incremental value of upper endoscopy for triage of patients with acute non-variceal upper-GI hemorrhage. Gastrointest Endosc 2004;60:9–14.

[95] Das A, Ben-Menachem T, Cooper GS, et al. Prediction of outcome in acute lower-gastrointestinal haemorrhage based on an artificial neural network: internal and external validation of a predictive model. Lancet 2003;362:1261–6.

[96] Targownik L, Gralnek IM. A risk score to predict need for treatment for upper GI hemorrhage. Gastrointest Endosc 2001;54:797–9.

[97] Chak A, Cooper GS, Lloyd LE, et al. Effectiveness of endoscopy in patients admitted to the intensive care unit with upper GI hemorrhage. Gastrointest Endosc 2001;53:6–13.

[98] Spiegel BM, Vakil NB, Ofman JJ. Endoscopy for acute nonvariceal upper gastrointestinal tract hemorrhage: is sooner better? A systematic review. Arch Intern Med 2001;161: 1393–404.

[99] Lee JG, Turnipseed S, Romano PS, et al. Endoscopy-based triage significantly reduces hospitalization rates and costs of treating upper GI bleeding: a randomized controlled trial. Gastrointest Endosc 1999;50:755–61.

[100] Bjorkman DJ, Zaman A, Fennerty MB, et al. Urgent vs. elective endoscopy for acute nonvariceal upper-GI bleeding: an effectiveness study. Gastrointest Endosc 2004;60:1–8.

[101] Kovacs TO, Jensen DM. Recent advances in the endoscopic diagnosis and therapy of upper gastrointestinal, small intestinal, and colonic bleeding. Med Clin North Am 2002;86:1319–56.

[102] Kogan FJ, Sampliner RE, Feldshon SD, et al. The yield of diagnostic upper endoscopy: results of a prospective audit. J Clin Gastroenterol 1985;7:488–91.

[103] Kahn KL, Kosecoff J, Chassin MR, et al. The use and misuse of upper gastrointestinal endoscopy. Ann Intern Med 1988;109:664–70.

[104] Clarke GA, Jacobson BC, Hammett RJ, et al. The indications, utilization and safety of gastrointestinal endoscopy in an extremely elderly patient cohort. Endoscopy 2001;33: 580–4.

[105] Hawkey GM, Cole AT, McIntyre AS, et al. Drug treatments in upper gastrointestinal bleeding: value of endoscopic findings as surrogate end points. Gut 2001;49:372–9.

[106] Lau JY, Sung JJ, Chan AC, et al. Stigmata of hemorrhage in bleeding peptic ulcers: an interobserver agreement study among international experts. Gastrointest Endosc 1997;46: 33–6.

[107] Mondardini A, Barletti C, Rocca G, et al. Non-variceal upper gastrointestinal bleeding and Forrest's classification: diagnostic agreement between endoscopists from the same area. Endoscopy 1998;30:508–12.

[108] Swain P. What should be done when initial endoscopic therapy for bleeding peptic ulcer fails? Endoscopy 1995;27:321–8.

[109] Jensen DM, Kovacs TO, Jutabha R, et al. Randomized trial of medical or endoscopic therapy to prevent recurrent ulcer hemorrhage in patients with adherent clots. Gastroenterology 2002;123:407–13.

[110] Marmo R, Rotondano G, Bianco MA, et al. Outcome of endoscopic treatment for peptic ulcer bleeding: is a second look necessary? A meta-analysis. Gastrointest Endosc 2003;57:62–7.

[111] Spiegel BM, Ofman JJ, Woods K, et al. Minimizing recurrent peptic ulcer hemorrhage after endoscopic hemostasis: the cost-effectiveness of competing strategies. Am J Gastroenterol 2003;98:86–97.

[112] Fullarton GM, Murray WR. Prediction of rebleeding in peptic ulcers by visual stigmata and endoscopic Doppler ultrasound criteria. Endoscopy 1990;22:68–71.

[113] Lee YT, Chan FK, Ng EK, et al. EUS-guided injection of cyanoacrylate for bleeding gastric varices. Gastrointest Endosc 2000;52:168–74.

[114] Konishi Y, Nakamura T, Kida H, et al. Catheter US probe EUS evaluation of gastric cardia and perigastric vascular structures to predict esophageal variceal recurrence. Gastrointest Endosc 2002;55:197–203.

[115] Lai L, Poneros J, Santilli J, et al. EUS-guided portal vein catheterization and pressure measurement in an animal model: a pilot study of feasibility. Gastrointest Endosc 2004;59: 280–3.

[116] Cattan P, Cuillerier E, Cellier C, et al. Hemobilia caused by a pseudoaneurysm of the hepatic artery diagnosed by EUS. Gastrointest Endosc 1999;49:252–5.

[117] Ribeiro A, Vazquez-Sequeiros E, Wiersema MJ. Doppler EUS-guided treatment of gastric Dieulafoy's lesion. Gastrointest Endosc 2001;53:807–9.

[118] Wong RC, Chak A, Kobayashi K, et al. Role of Doppler US in acute peptic ulcer hemor-rhage: can it predict failure of endoscopic therapy? Gastrointest Endosc 2000;52: 315–21.

[119] Fraser GM, Rankin RN, Cummack DH. Radiology and endoscopy in acute upper gastro-intestinal bleeding. BMJ 1976;1:270–1.

[120] Op den Orth JO. Use of barium in evaluation of disorders of the upper gastrointestinal tract: current status. Radiology 1989;173:601–8.

[121] Lewis BS. Radiology versus endoscopy of the small bowel. Gastrointest Endosc Clin N Am 1999;9:13–27.

[122] Lo SK. Capsule endoscopy in the diagnosis and management of inflammatory bowel dis-ease. Gastrointest Endosc Clin N Am 2004;14:179–93.

[123] Kovacs TO. Small bowel bleeding. Curr Treat Options Gastroenterol 2005;8:31–8.

Gastroenterol Clin N Am 34 (2005) 607–621

GASTROENTEROLOGY CLINICS
OF NORTH AMERICA

ELSEVIER
SAUNDERS

Nonvariceal Upper Gastrointestinal Bleeding: Standard and New Treatment

Charles B Ferguson, MB, Robert M. Mitchell, MB*

Department of Gastroenterology, Belfast City Hospital, Lisburn Road, Belfast BT9 7AB, Northern Ireland

Nonvariceal upper gastrointestinal bleeding (UGIB) remains a common emergency for gastroenterologists with an annual incidence of 50 to 150 per 100,000 of the population. Mortality from UGIB is around 10%, and may reach 35% in patients hospitalized with another medical condition. Serious comorbidity remains an independent risk factor for UGIB mortality, which is often attributable to increasing age and associated illnesses [1]. A recent time trend analysis by a Dutch group has demonstrated a decrease in incidence of UGIB (from 61.7 per 100,000 per year in 1993–1994 to 47 per 100,000 per year in 2000), but has not demonstrated a reduction in mortality or rebleeding rates [2], even though there have been significant advances in medical and endoscopic management of serious UGIB. An ageing population with potentially serious comorbidities helps to explain the lack of concordance between the overall population incidence and mortality rate for UGIB. Patients over 80 years of age now account for around 25% of all UGIB and 33% of UGIB occurring in hospitalized patients [1].

ETIOLOGY OF NONVARICEAL UPPER GASTROINTESTINAL BLEEDING

The causes and historically quoted frequencies of nonvariceal UGIB are shown in Table 1. There is controversy regarding the relative contribution of peptic ulcer bleeding to overall UGIB rates. Recent data from the Clinical Outcome Research Initiative suggest that the frequency of peptic ulcer as a cause of UGIB may have been overestimated. In 7822 endoscopies performed for UGIB, peptic ulcer was the likely cause in only 1610 patients (20.6%) [3]. Data from the Canadian Registry on Nonvariceal Upper Gastrointestinal Bleeding and Endoscopy, however, identified peptic ulcers in 50% of patients presenting to community and tertiary care institutions between 1999 and 2002 [4]. Regardless of the historical frequency of peptic ulcer bleeding, the

*Corresponding author. E-mail address: michael.mitchell@bch.n-i.nhs.uk (R.M. Mitchell).

0889-8553/05/$ – see front matter
doi:10.1016/j.gtc.2005.08.003

Table 1
Causes of nonvariceal upper gastrointestinal bleeding

Diagnosis	Incidence (%)
Peptic ulcer	30–50
Mallory-Weiss tear	15–20
Erosive gastritis or duodenitis	10–15
Esophagitis	5–10
Malignancy	1–2
Angiodysplasia or vascular malformations	5
Other	5

incidence of peptic ulcer disease should decline with more widespread *Helicobacter pylori* eradication. In addition, widespread use of cyclooxygenase-2–specific nonsteroidal anti-inflammatory drugs may also affect peptic ulcer risk, although prescription of this particular class of drugs worldwide has been severely affected by recent statements by the US Food and Drug Administration and other national drug monitoring organizations.

CLINICAL RISK ASSESSMENT

One of the major challenges of managing UGIB involves identifying patients who are at high risk of rebleeding and death; conversely, identifying patients who are suitable for early discharge and outpatient endoscopy is also important for effective resource use. Several clinical scoring systems have been developed to help predict outcome for patients with a view to improving patient management and promoting cost-effective use of resources. In most published scoring systems, a combination of clinical, laboratory, and endoscopic variables are weighted to produce a score that predicts the risk of mortality, recurrent hemorrhage, need for clinical intervention, or suitability for early discharge. The most commonly used systems (Rockall score, the Baylor bleeding score, the Cedars-Sinai Medical Centre Predictive Index, and the Blatchford score) were recently excellently reviewed by Das and Wong [5]. Several factors are associated with poor outcome from UGIB and may be related to the patient's presentation and comorbidities, or to the behavior of the ulcer:

Shock
Melena
Anemia at presentation
Significant fresh blood in vomit, gastric aspirate, or rectum
Concurrent sepsis
General poor health
Liver, renal, cardiac disease
Large ulcer size
Persistent bleeding despite endoscopic therapy
Recurrent bleeding

Inclusion of endoscopic stigmata of recent hemorrhage (SRH) that relate to increased risk of rebleeding and death into scoring systems increases the sensitivity for predicting patients at high or low risk of adverse events compared with nonendoscopic assessments [6,7]. In addition, early endoscopy-based triage (within 12 hours of admission) may allow safe and early discharge of low-risk patients with no increased rate of rebleeding or mortality [8]. Risk stratification using nonendoscopic parameters has the advantage that it can be performed readily on initial presentation in the emergency department, however, and if early endoscopy, which requires skilled staff and resources, is not available, appropriate initial risk assessment can be made. Clearly, more studies are required to clarify the role of endoscopy in early risk assessment. More generally, care must be taken when applying a risk stratification scoring system to any patient population not represented by the original studies, because racial, cultural, or ethnic factors may affect a populations' risk [9].

INITIAL MANAGEMENT

Resuscitation and optimization of comorbid conditions are vital in the initial management of patients before endoscopy. Transfusion of blood and blood products may be necessary and patients often require management in an intensive care setting. Endotracheal intubation remains controversial in significant nonvariceal UGIB. The endoscopist's task is made easier and the risk of massive aspiration in a patient with reduced level of consciousness is reduced if a patient is intubated; however, evidence of a reduction in acquired pneumonia or cardiopulmonary events is lacking [10,11]. The presence of blood-stained nasogastric aspirate can be used to predict the presence of high-risk lesions and nasogastric tube insertion should be considered for some patients [12]. The optimum timing of endoscopy remains a balance between clinical need and resources, but endoscopy performed within 24 hours of hospital admission has been shown to reduce the length of hospital stay and may reduce the likelihood of rebleeding or surgical intervention in the highest risk patients [13].

ENDOSCOPIC ASSESSMENT

Endoscopic SRH [14] associated with a higher risk of rebleeding, surgical intervention, and death have been well defined. High-risk lesions, such as actively bleeding ulcers, nonbleeding visible vessels (NBVV), and adherent clots [15], require aggressive intervention because ulcer rebleeding is associated with a 5- to 16-fold increase in mortality [16], and effective endoscopic management can substantially reduce this risk. The rebleeding rate of ulcers with a clean base or red or blue spots is low [17,18], and endoscopic intervention is usually not recommended [9].

Although actively bleeding vessels are consistently identified by endoscopists, this is not the case for other SRH, particularly NBVV and flat pigmented spots [19]. Attention has turned to alternative approaches to assess lesions more objectively. Doppler examination of ulcers was assessed as a means of obtaining objective evidence of rebleeding risk in 100 patients admitted with UGIB but not bleeding at the time of index endoscopy. Doppler findings were compared with the Forrest classification of the ulcer [20]. Ulcers were assessed for the presence of blood vessels and were considered to be Doppler-positive if a vessel no deeper than 1 mm was identified. Doppler-positive ulcers and those in the Forrest group with adherent clot or visible vessels were treated endoscopically. There was agreement between the Forrest classification and Doppler in only 58% of cases. Rebleeding, requirement for surgery, and mortality rate were all significantly lower in the Doppler-assessed group. The authors suggest that Doppler assessment can guide appropriate endoscopic intervention for patients with NBVV. Technical and resource limitations, however, mean this technique is unlikely to be widely available for some time.

Not infrequently, excessive blood in the upper gastrointestinal tract may preclude an accurate endoscopic diagnosis. A retrospective study by Cheng and coworkers [21] identified 25 of (1.7%) 1459 patients where a diagnosis could not be made endoscopically because of blood obscuring the examination field. Not surprisingly, these patients had a significantly higher rate of complications, rebleeding, need for surgery, and mortality. The authors stress the importance of good preparation along with the removal of blood during the procedure. Bolus administration of intravenous erythromycin before endoscopy has been shown to clear the stomach of blood, thereby increasing the likelihood of successful hemostasis and reducing the need for further interventions [22,23].

ENDOSCOPIC MANAGEMENT

Endoscopic intervention is beneficial in high-risk patients with UGIB, reducing the rate of rebleeding, need for surgical intervention, and mortality [24]. It is likely that most hemostatic techniques are equally effective when used alone. Recent research has focused on the role of combination therapies and newer mechanical means of homeostasis. Most of the following text refers to peptic ulcer bleeding but may be applicable in other causes of nonvariceal UGIB.

Injection Therapy

Injection of dilute (1:10,000) adrenaline in 1-mL aliquots around the bleeding points results in hemostasis in up to 100% of patients with bleeding peptic ulcers, probably by a combination of vascular tamponade and vasoconstriction, with a concomitant reduction in rebleeding rates from 40% to 15% [25,26]. The dose of adrenaline required to achieve hemostasis is probably dependent on the individual patient; however, in a study of 156 patients with Forrest type I or IIa lesions a larger volume (13–20 versus 5–10 mL) resulted in less rebleeding (15.4% versus 30.8%) [27]. Although injection with adrenaline is successful in achieving initial hemostasis, the published rebleed rates of 15% to 36% remains relatively high [28,29]. Attention has focused on alternative techniques (eg, heat or mechanical) or combination therapy to determine if there is any additional benefit.

Sclerosants, such as ethanol, polidocanol, and ethanolamine, have been used to promote vessel thrombosis, but evidence to date suggests these agents are no better, and may have more risk, than adrenaline [28,30–32]. In one study, ethanol injection alone was shown to have a rebleeding rate as low as 4% [33];

however, most other published studies have demonstrated similar or worse rates of hemostasis than adrenaline alone. A combination of adrenaline and ethanol may improve hemostasis and shorten duration of hospital stay for patients with spurting hemorrhage [31].

Thrombin-fibrinogen mixture (fibrin-sealant glue) does not seem to confer any additional benefit beyond adrenaline alone when used in a one-off basis in combination with adrenaline injection for patients with high-risk peptic ulcers, although it may be of particular use in patients with active bleeding [34]. A study involving 51 patients with active bleeding or NBVV demonstrated lower rebleeding rates with a single treatment with combination adrenaline and fibrin sealant compared with adrenaline alone, although there was no difference in mortality, transfusion requirements, surgery, or duration of hospital stay [35]. Repeated injection of fibrin glue following treatment with dilute adrenaline in patients with active bleeding or NBVV was subsequently compared with single application of fibrin glue or polidocanol following adrenaline injection. Patients underwent daily endoscopy until the ulcer base was clean or covered in hematin. Patients in the repeat treatment group had significantly higher rates of hemostasis with less rebleeding compared with the polidocanol group, although mortality rates were not reduced [36]. The major drawback of this schedule is the cost incurred by repeated daily procedures. In another study, endoscopic intervention with a combination of adrenaline injection and 600 to 1000 IU human thrombin has been shown to be more effective than injection of adrenaline alone, with a reduction in rebleeding (4.5% versus 20%), transfusion requirement, and mortality [37].

Injection with *N*-butyl-2-cyanoacrylate has been shown to be effective for control of variceal bleeding [38], but its role in nonvariceal UGIB remains uncertain. In a small study of 32 cases it was no more effective than injection with dilute adrenaline for control of bleeding ulcers [28]. More recently, Lee and coworkers [39] showed significantly lower rebleeding rate for patients with Forrest type Ia lesions treated with *N*-butyl-2-cyanoacrylate compared with injection with hypertonic saline-adrenaline injection. There was no overall benefit in the use of *N*-butyl-2-cyanoacrylate with regards to hemostasis rates, emergency surgery, or mortality. Arterial embolization is a recognized complication of this treatment, and occurred in 2 of 63 patients in the treatment group. The authors recommend *N*-butyl-2-cyanoacrylate injection only as a measure of last resort before surgery because of potentially fatal adverse effects.

Thermal Techniques

Several thermal techniques have been used for the control of nonvariceal UGIB. Homeostasis is achieved by compression of the artery during heating (coaption) and the effect of heat on tissue.

Noncontact thermal techniques

Laser (neodymium:yttrium-aluminum-garnet) and argon plasma coagulation are the only noncontact thermal therapies currently available. Argon plasma coagulation causes hemostasis by conducting a high-frequency electrical current through a beam of ionized argon gas, resulting in superficial tissue damage and coagulation. Although the technique is generally safe and relatively straightforward, the efficacy has yet to be fully determined. A prospective observational study into the use of argon plasma coagulation in 254 patients with nonvariceal UGIB revealed initial hemostasis rates of 75.9% and rebleeding rates of 5.7% with argon plasma coagulation alone [40]. When a second endoscopic technique was added, initial hemostasis was achieved in 99.6%. In the only comparative randomized trial involving argon plasma coagulation in nonvariceal UGIB, rates of hemostasis, rebleeding, emergency surgery, and 30-day mortality were comparable with the heater probe, although the numbers in this study (N = 41) were too small to detect a difference [41]. Chau and coworkers [42] compared combination treatment with adrenaline and heater probe with adrenaline and argon plasma coagulation in a prospective, randomized, controlled trial involving 185 patients with bleeding peptic ulcers. There was no significant difference in primary hemostasis, procedure duration, rebleeding, requirement for surgery, 30-day mortality, or ulcer healing at 8 weeks, suggesting that combination therapy with adrenaline and argon plasma coagulation is as effective as heater probe in high-risk patients with bleeding ulcers.

Laser therapy has been shown to be as effective as injection with epinephrine-polidocanol [43], but because of technical constraints of the technique, laser therapy is not routinely used in the management of nonvariceal UGIB.

Contact thermal techniques

Bipolar electrocoagulation and heater probe thermocoagulation use thermal contact to achieve hemostasis by compression of the vessel and coaption. A bipolar electrocoagulation device may include an injector-irrigator component (eg, Gold probe, Boston Scientific, Boston, MA) to allow injection of adrenaline and irrigation of the culprit lesion. Bipolar electrocoagulation has been shown to reduce the rebleeding rate when compared with normal saline injection in high-risk bleeding ulcers [44], and in combination with adrenaline in type IIb ulcers [45].

Combination therapy with heater probe thermocoagulation and adrenaline in the treatment of actively bleeding peptic ulcers resulted in hemostasis in up to 98.6%, with rebleeding in 8.2% [46]. In another study, however, there was no significant difference in rates of rebleeding, requirement for surgery, and length of hospital stay when compared with adrenaline alone [29]. Subgroup analysis, however, did illustrate benefit in patients with Forrest Ia lesions, with dual therapy resulting in significantly lower rebleeding rates and nonsignificant reductions in emergency surgery and length of hospital stay. When used alone, heater probe thermocoagulation was not superior to combination treatment with adrenaline and polidocanol in patients with Forrest type I, IIa, and IIb ulcers [47]. Heater probe thermocoagulation (HPC) in combination with thrombin was compared to HPC and placebo in 247 patients with bleeding peptic ulcers and was found to confer no benefit when compared with the placebo arm with regards to hemostasis, rebleeding rates, requirement for surgery, adverse events, or mortality [48].

Mechanical Techniques

Mechanical methods of achieving hemostasis are often used in variceal UGIB. Endoloops and particularly clips (eg, the Hemoclip [Teleflex Medical, Research Triangle Park, NC]), however, are likely to play an increasing role in the control of nonvariceal UGIB. Hemostasis using endoclips involves deployment of a clip to achieve vascular compression. So far the Hemoclip has been safe and effective, achieving homeostasis rates of up to 100% [49]. Comparative studies with other endoscopic techniques suggest lower rebleeding rates than adrenaline injection [50], ethanol [51], or hypertonic saline-epinephrine [52]. The additional benefit of adrenaline with a mechanical method is unclear [53]. A randomized comparative study of injection of epinephrine-polidocanol and Hemoclip versus Hemoclip alone, however, showed clipping to be inferior to combination Hemoclip–adrenaline injection therapy in the treatment of bleeding peptic ulcers [54]. Chung and coworkers [52] found the Hemoclip to be an effective method for hemostasis and safer than hypertonic saline-epinephrine, and combination treatment with injection therapy and Hemoclips was equivalent to either treatment alone for control of bleeding. Rebleeding rates and the need for surgery were higher, however, in the adrenaline group. A potential limitation of the Hemoclip is the technical difficulty in applying the clips to difficult-to-reach lesions, particularly those high on the gastric lesser curve or posterior wall of the duodenum. This was demonstrated in a comparative study of Hemoclip with heater probe thermocoagulation in which the overall rates of hemostasis were 85% and 100%, respectively. In the subgroup of difficult-to-approach lesions the homeostasis rate fell to 30% and 82%, respectively. Rotatable and more versatile endoclips may help to lessen this problem. In addition, devices that can deploy multiple or stronger clips are needed. Two small studies have evaluated the role of Hemoclips for control of bleeding caused by Dieulafoy's lesion. Hemostasis was generally successful and there was a trend toward reduction in the need for repeat procedures [55,56].

Endoscopic band ligation is currently technically easier to use than endoclips and has been shown to be safe and effective for control of small lesions in 19 patients with acute peptic ulcer bleeding [57]. Rubber band ligation has recently been assessed in a small group of patients with UGIB secondary to Dieulafoy's lesion and found to be as effective as injection with or without thermal therapy [58].

Adherent Clots

Special mention needs to be made regarding the problem of adherent clots. A subgroup analysis of patients with adherent clots in early endoscopic studies demonstrated little or no benefit of endoscopic therapy for ulcers with adherent clots [59–62]. A subsequent meta-analysis showed significant benefit only in patients with active bleeding or NBVV [24]. A randomized controlled trial to assess endoscopic intervention in patients with severe UGIB and adherent clot randomized 32 patients to medical or combination therapy following irrigation of the clot [45]. Endoscopic therapy consisted of adrenaline injection, shaving of the clot with cold guillotine, and bipolar coagulation of the under-lying stigmata. Combination therapy was shown to be safe with significantly less early rebleeding compared with medical therapy, although the small sample size, unexpectedly low rebleed rates in the treatment group (0%), and unequal distribution of confounding factors in the two groups means that caution needs to be taken when extrapolating the results. In addition, various studies have shown intraobserver variation in the labeling of SRH, and the degree of clot adherence may vary depending on the extent of clot irrigation [63,64]. For instance, in one study 5 minutes of irrigation by a bipolar probe was found to remove clot in 43% of patients, whereas irrigation with a syringe only removed 9% of the clot [65]. In another study, 10 seconds of irrigation with WaterPik (Teledyne, Fort Collins, CO) removed clots in a further 26% of patients [66]. Placement of a newly designed transparent irrigating hood that allows forceful irrigation yet maintains a reasonable endoscopic view may prove useful for clot removal. Early experience suggests that total procedure time may be reduced when using this device [67,68]. Although the optimum technique for clot removal is unclear, the value of clot removal is clear, because high-risk SRH may be exposed in the underlying ulcer in a further 30% of patients. Rebleeding rates for untreated ulcers with adherent clot are reported as 20% and in the group where clots remained was 8%,which is similar to that expected in low-risk lesions, such as flat pigmented spots [15]. Current practice among experienced endoscopists involves targeted irrigation of an adherent clot to dislodge it, if possible, followed by treatment of the underlying lesion [45].

SECOND-LOOK ENDOSCOPY AND ENDOSCOPIC RETREATMENT

Several studies investigating the role of routine second-look endoscopy following endoscopic treatment have shown no benefit with regards to clinically significant outcomes for unselected patient populations [69], although there may be a role in high-risk patients [70,71]. Repeat endoscopy is indicated if there is clinical evidence of rebleeding or if the initial procedure was unsuccessful or partially successful, although this depends on local endoscopic and surgical expertise [9,72]. In expert centers, endoscopic retreatment is associated with fewer complications, less need for surgery, and no increased mortality risk compared with surgery [73].

FUTURE DIRECTIONS IN ENDOSCOPY
Endoscopic Suturing

A variety of endoscopic suturing devices have been developed primarily for gastroplication in patients with gastroesophageal reflux. Endoscopic suturing for UGIB is an attractive prospect, but further development of new devices is required before suturing for UGIB can be widely adopted. Such issues as the device size and maneuverability, and precise control of suture depth, need to be addressed.

Cryotherapy

Application of heat to bleeding or potentially bleeding lesions has drawbacks, such as the requirement for contact, expense, lack of control of depth of injury, and difficulty in treating multiple or diffuse lesions. Cryosurgery involves freezing tissue to achieve a therapeutic response. Gastric freezing to achieve hemostasis during variceal and nonvariceal bleeding has been possible for several decades, although evidence of therapeutic benefit from the original techniques was lacking [74]. More recently, delivery systems for liquid nitrogen or nitrous oxide have made endoscopic cryotherapy possible for bleeding and other applications [75–77]. Delivery of nitrous oxide to result in cryotherapy relies on the Joule-Thompson effect: rapid expansion of compressed gas results in a drop in temperature of the gas. This allows noncontact therapy to localized or diffuse vascular lesions. The technique remains experimental, but it seem to be safe and effective for radiation proctitis and vascular malformations, and there may be potential use in other gastrointestinal vascular lesions.

PROTON PUMP INHIBITORS

In vitro studies of the effect of gastric pH on platelet aggregation and coagulation provide the rationale for acid suppression in UGIB. If gastric pH is maintained above pH6 (by infusional proton pump inhibitors), platelet aggregation is optimized and fibrinolysis relatively inhibited, thereby potentially improving the likelihood of clot stability at an ulcer site. Individual trials of H_2 receptor antagonists have generally failed to demonstrate a clinical benefit in UGIB [78,79], although a meta-analysis has suggested a weak effect [80]. Several studies have evaluated intravenous proton pump inhibitors for nonvariceal UGIB; unfortunately, these trials are heterogeneous in terms of patient population, regimen of proton pump inhibitor, and timing or type of endoscopic intervention, making comparisons difficult. Five meta-analyses of proton pump inhibitors in nonvariceal UGIB have now shown a benefit, however, in terms of rebleeding and need for surgery, but not for mortality [81–85]. The usual intravenous regime for omeprazole therapy in the more robust studies was an 80-mg intravenous bolus of omeprazole followed by a continuous infusion of 8 mg/h for up to 72 hours. This regimen resulted in a reduction of rebleeding from 22.5% to 6.7%, representing a number needed to treat (NNT) of 6 to prevent one person bleeding within 30 days [84]. Subsequent studies using lower intravenous doses of omeprazole [86] or high-dose oral omeprazole [87–89] also demonstrated a reduction in rebleeding rate. Further study is required to determine the optimum dose and schedule of proton pump inhibitors in UGIB. It seems reasonable, however, to treat patients with high-risk SRH with intravenous or high-dose oral proton pump inhibitors after endoscopic therapy has been administered.

SUMMARY

Nonvariceal UGIB remains a significant cause of morbidity and mortality. Many patients require intensive supportive therapy and aggressive management of medical comorbidities. Age and concurrent medical conditions remain

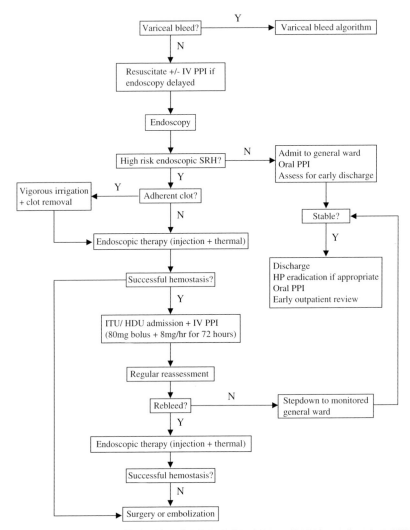

Fig. 1. Algorithm for management of nonvariceal UGIB. HDU, high dependency unit; HP, *Helicobacter pylori*; ITU, intensive therapy unit; IV, intravenous; PPI, proton pump inhibitor; SRH, stigmata of recent hemorrhage.

major determinants of morbidity. Most UGIB stops spontaneously. Appropriate therapy for patients who continue to bleed, or in patients who rebleed after initial hemostasis has been achieved, includes aggressive endoscopy, usually with a combination of thermal and injection therapy, followed by intravenous or high-dose oral proton pump inhibitor. Mechanical endoscopic devices are promising for achieving hemostasis in peptic ulcer bleeding. Patients at high risk of rebleeding can usually be identified by clinical and endoscopic means and treated appropriately.

The algorithm used for management of nonvariceal UGIB at the authors' institution is summarized in Fig. 1. It is their policy to include gastroenterologists, intensive care physicians, surgeons, and radiologists at an early stage of the admission and decision- making process to optimize care of potentially ill patients. The value of regular and repeated clinical assessment, adequate resuscitation, and appropriate multidisciplinary input cannot be overstated.

References

[1] Rockall TA, Logan RF, Devlin HB, et al. Incidence of and mortality from acute upper gastrointestinal haemorrhage in the United Kingdom. Steering Committee and members of the National Audit of Acute Upper Gastrointestinal Haemorrhage. BMJ 1995;311:222–6.

[2] van Leerdam ME, Vreeburg EM, Rauws EA, et al. Acute upper GI bleeding: did anything change? Time trend analysis of incidence and outcome of acute upper GI bleeding between 1993/1994 and 2000. Am J Gastroenterol 2003;98:1494–9.

[3] Boonpongmanee S, Fleischer DE, Pezzullo JC, et al. The frequency of peptic ulcer as a cause of upper-GI bleeding is exaggerated. Gastrointest Endosc 2004;59:788–94.

[4] Barkun A, Sabbah S, Enns R, et al. The Canadian Registry on Nonvariceal Upper Gastrointestinal Bleeding and Endoscopy (RUGBE): endoscopic hemostasis and proton pump inhibition are associated with improved outcomes in a real-life setting. Am J Gastroenterol 2004;99:1238–46.

[5] Das A, Wong RC. Prediction of outcome of acute GI hemorrhage: a review of risk scores and predictive models. Gastrointest Endosc 2004;60:85–93.

[6] Gralnek IM, Dulai GS. Incremental value of upper endoscopy for triage of patients with acute non-variceal upper-GI hemorrhage. Gastrointest Endosc 2004;60:9–14.

[7] Blatchford O, Murray WR, Blatchford M. A risk score to predict need for treatment for upper-gastrointestinal haemorrhage. Lancet 2000;356:1318–21.

[8] Hay JA, Maldonado L, Weingarten SR, et al. Prospective evaluation of a clinical guideline recommending hospital length of stay in upper gastrointestinal tract hemorrhage. JAMA 1997;278:2151–6.

[9] Barkun A, Bardou M, Marshall JK. Consensus recommendations for managing patients with nonvariceal upper gastrointestinal bleeding. Ann Intern Med 2003;139:843–57.

[10] Lipper B, Simon D, Cerrone F. Pulmonary aspiration during emergency endoscopy in patients with upper gastrointestinal hemorrhage. Crit Care Med 1991;19:330–3.

[11] Rudolph SJ, Landsverk BK, Freeman ML. Endotracheal intubation for airway protection during endoscopy for severe upper GI hemorrhage. Gastrointest Endosc 2003;57:58–61.

[12] Aljebreen AM, Fallone CA, Barkun AN. Nasogastric aspirate predicts high-risk endoscopic lesions in patients with acute upper-GI bleeding. Gastrointest Endosc 2004;59:172–8.

[13] Cooper GS, Chak A, Way LE, et al. Early endoscopy in upper gastrointestinal hemorrhage: associations with recurrent bleeding, surgery, and length of hospital stay. Gastrointest Endosc 1999;49:145–52.

[14] Forrest JA, Finlayson ND, Shearman DJ. Endoscopy in gastrointestinal bleeding. Lancet 1974;2:394–7.

[15] Laine L, Peterson WL. Bleeding peptic ulcer. N Engl J Med 1994;331:717–27.

[16] Rockall TA, Logan RF, Devlin HB, et al. Risk assessment after acute upper gastrointestinal haemorrhage. Gut 1996;38:316–21.

[17] Palmer KR. Ulcers and nonvariceal bleeding. Endoscopy 2000;32:118–23.

[18] Bornman PC, Theodorou NA, Shuttleworth RD, et al. Importance of hypovolaemic shock and endoscopic signs in predicting recurrent haemorrhage from peptic ulceration: a prospective evaluation. BMJ 1985;291:245–7.

[19] Mondardini A, Barletti C, Rocca G, et al. Non-variceal upper gastrointestinal bleeding and Forrest's classification: diagnostic agreement between endoscopists from the same area. Endoscopy 1998;30:508–12.

[20] Kohler B, Maier M, Benz C, et al. Acute ulcer bleeding: a prospective randomized trial to compare Doppler and Forrest classifications in endoscopic diagnosis and therapy. Dig Dis Sci 1997;42:1370–4.

[21] Cheng CL, Lee CS, Liu NJ, et al. Overlooked lesions at emergency endoscopy for acute nonvariceal upper gastrointestinal bleeding. Endoscopy 2002;34:527–30.

[22] Coffin B, Pocard M, Panis Y, et al. Erythromycin improves the quality of EGD in patients with acute upper GI bleeding: a randomized controlled study. Gastrointest Endosc 2002;56: 174–9.

[23] Frossard JL, Spahr L, Queneau PE, et al. Erythromycin intravenous bolus infusion in acute upper gastrointestinal bleeding: a randomized, controlled, double-blind trial. Gastroenterology 2002;123:17–23.

[24] Cook DJ, Guyatt GH, Salena BJ, et al. Endoscopic therapy for acute nonvariceal upper gastrointestinal hemorrhage: a meta-analysis. Gastroenterology 1992;102:139–48.

[25] Chung SC, Leung JW, Steele RJ, et al. Endoscopic injection of adrenaline for actively bleeding ulcers: a randomised trial. BMJ 1988;296:1631–3.

[26] Ogra R, Lane M, Wong P, et al. Endoscopic injection therapy for non-variceal upper gastrointestinal bleeding at Auckland Hospital. N Z Med J 2002;115:U255.

[27] Lin HJ, Hsieh YH, Tseng GY, et al. A prospective, randomized trial of large- versus small-volume endoscopic injection of epinephrine for peptic ulcer bleeding. Gastrointest Endosc 2002;55:615–9.

[28] Choudari CP, Palmer KR. Endoscopic injection therapy for bleeding peptic ulcer; a comparison of adrenaline alone with adrenaline plus ethanolamine oleate. Gut 1994;35: 608–10.

[29] Chung SS, Lau JY, Sung JJ, et al. Randomised comparison between adrenaline injection alone and adrenaline injection plus heat probe treatment for actively bleeding ulcers. BMJ 1997;314:1307–11.

[30] Chung SC, Leong HT, Chan AC, et al. Epinephrine or epinephrine plus alcohol for injection of bleeding ulcers: a prospective randomized trial. Gastrointest Endosc 1996;43:591–5.

[31] Lin HJ, Perng CL, Lee SD. Is sclerosant injection mandatory after an epinephrine injection for arrest of peptic ulcer haemorrhage? A prospective, randomised, comparative study. Gut 1993;34:1182–5.

[32] Villanueva C, Balanzo J, Espinos JC, et al. Endoscopic injection therapy of bleeding ulcer: a prospective and randomized comparison of adrenaline alone or with polidocanol. J Clin Gastroenterol 1993;17:195–200.

[33] Asaki S. Efficacy of endoscopic pure ethanol injection method for gastrointestinal ulcer bleeding. World J Surg 2000;24:294–8.

[34] Pescatore P, Jornod P, Borovicka J, et al. Epinephrine versus epinephrine plus fibrin glue injection in peptic ulcer bleeding: a prospective randomized trial. Gastrointest Endosc 2002;55:348–53.

[35] Lin HJ, Hsieh YH, Tseng GY, et al. Endoscopic injection with fibrin sealant versus epinephrine for arrest of peptic ulcer bleeding: a randomized, comparative trial. J Clin Gastroenterol 2002;35:218–21.

[36] Rutgeerts P, Rauws E, Wara P, et al. Randomised trial of single and repeated fibrin glue compared with injection of polidocanol in treatment of bleeding peptic ulcer. Lancet 1997;350: 692–6.

[37] Kubba AK, Murphy W, Palmer KR. Endoscopic injection for bleeding peptic ulcer: a comparison of adrenaline alone with adrenaline plus human thrombin. Gastroenterology 1996;111:623–8.

[38] Binmoeller KF, Soehendra N. Superglue: the answer to variceal bleeding and fundal varices? Endoscopy 1995;27:392–6.

[39] Lee KJ, Kim JH, Hahm KB, et al. Randomized trial of N-butyl-2-cyanoacrylate compared with injection of hypertonic saline-epinephrine in the endoscopic treatment of bleeding peptic ulcers. Endoscopy 2000;32:505–11.

[40] Kanai M, Hamada A, Endo Y, et al. Efficacy of argon plasma coagulation in nonvariceal upper gastrointestinal bleeding. Endoscopy 2004;36:1085–8.

[41] Cipolletta L, Bianco MA, Rotondano G, et al. Prospective comparison of argon plasma coagulator and heater probe in the endoscopic treatment of major peptic ulcer bleeding. Gastrointest Endosc 1998;48:191–5.

[42] Chau CH, Siu WT, Law BK, et al. Randomized controlled trial comparing epinephrine injection plus heat probe coagulation versus epinephrine injection plus argon plasma coagulation for bleeding peptic ulcers. Gastrointest Endosc 2003;57:455–61.

[43] Rutgeerts P, Vantrappen G, Broeckaert L, et al. Comparison of endoscopic polidocanol injection and YAG laser therapy for bleeding peptic ulcers. Lancet 1989;1:1164–7.

[44] Laine L, Estrada R. Randomized trial of normal saline solution injection versus bipolar electrocoagulation for treatment of patients with high-risk bleeding ulcers: is local tamponade enough? Gastrointest Endosc 2002;55:6–10.

[45] Jensen DM, Kovacs TO, Jutabha R, et al. Randomized trial of medical or endoscopic therapy to prevent recurrent ulcer hemorrhage in patients with adherent clots. Gastroenterology 2002;123:407–13.

[46] Wong SK, Yu LM, Lau JY, et al. Prediction of therapeutic failure after adrenaline injection plus heater probe treatment in patients with bleeding peptic ulcer. Gut 2002;50:322–5.

[47] Llach J, Bordas JM, Salmeron JM, et al. A prospective randomized trial of heater probe thermocoagulation versus injection therapy in peptic ulcer hemorrhage. Gastrointest Endosc 1996;43(2 Pt 1):117–20.

[48] Church NI, Dallal HJ, Masson J, et al. A randomized trial comparing heater probe plus thrombin with heater probe plus placebo for bleeding peptic ulcer. Gastroenterology 2003;125:396–403.

[49] Chou YC, Hsu PI, Lai KH, et al. A prospective, randomized trial of endoscopic hemoclip placement and distilled water injection for treatment of high-risk bleeding ulcers. Gastrointest Endosc 2003;57:324–8.

[50] Nagasu N, DiPalma JA. Bleeding ulcer: inject or clip? Am J Gastroenterol 1998;93:1998.

[51] Nagayama K, Tazawa J, Sakai Y, et al. Efficacy of endoscopic clipping for bleeding gastroduodenal ulcer: comparison with topical ethanol injection. Am J Gastroenterol 1999;94:2897–901.

[52] Chung IK, Ham JS, Kim HS, et al. Comparison of the hemostatic efficacy of the endoscopic hemoclip method with hypertonic saline-epinephrine injection and a combination of the two for the management of bleeding peptic ulcers. Gastrointest Endosc 1999;49:13–8.

[53] Buffoli F, Graffeo M, Nicosia F, et al. Peptic ulcer bleeding: comparison of two hemostatic procedures. Am J Gastroenterol 2001;96:89–94.

[54] Gevers AM, De Goede E, Simoens M, et al. A randomized trial comparing injection therapy with hemoclip and with injection combined with hemoclip for bleeding ulcers. Gastrointest Endosc 2002;55:466–9.

[55] Park CH, Sohn YH, Lee WS, et al. The usefulness of endoscopic hemoclipping for bleeding Dieulafoy lesions. Endoscopy 2003;35:388–92.

[56] Yamaguchi Y, Yamato T, Katsumi N, et al. Short-term and long-term benefits of endoscopic hemoclip application for Dieulafoy's lesion in the upper GI tract. Gastrointest Endosc 2003;57:653–6.

[57] Park CH, Lee WS, Joo YE, et al. Endoscopic band ligation for control of acute peptic ulcer bleeding. Endoscopy 2004;36:79–82.

[58] Mumtaz R, Shaukat M, Ramirez FC. Outcomes of endoscopic treatment of gastroduodenal Dieulafoy's lesion with rubber band ligation and thermal/injection therapy. J Clin Gastroenterol 2003;36:310–4.

[59] Swain CP, Bown SG, Storey DW, et al. Controlled trial of argon laser photocoagulation in bleeding peptic ulcers. Lancet 1981;2:1313–6.

[60] Swain CP, Kirkham JS, Salmon PR, et al. Controlled trial of Nd-YAG laser photocoagulation in bleeding peptic ulcers. Lancet 1986;1:1113–7.

[61] Balanzo J, Sainz S, Such J, et al. Endoscopic hemostasis by local injection of epinephrine and polidocanol in bleeding ulcer: a prospective randomized trial. Endoscopy 1988;20: 289–91.

[62] Matthewson K, Swain CP, Bland M, et al. Randomized comparison of Nd YAG laser, heater probe, and no endoscopic therapy for bleeding peptic ulcers. Gastroenterology 1990; 98(5 Pt 1):1239–44.

[63] Laine L, Freeman M, Cohen H. Lack of uniformity in evaluation of endoscopic prognostic features of bleeding ulcers. Gastrointest Endosc 1994;40:411–7.

[64] Lau JY, Sung JJ, Chan AC, et al. Stigmata of hemorrhage in bleeding peptic ulcers: an interobserver agreement study among international experts. Gastrointest Endosc 1997;46: 33–6.

[65] Laine L, Stein C, Sharma V. A prospective outcome study of patients with clot in an ulcer and the effect of irrigation. Gastrointest Endosc 1996;43(2 Pt 1):107–10.

[66] Lin HJ, Wang K, Perng CL, et al. Natural history of bleeding peptic ulcers with a tightly adherent blood clot: a prospective observation. Gastrointest Endosc 1996;43:470–3.

[67] Kume K, Yoshikawa I, Otsuki M. Endoscopic treatment of upper GI hemorrhage with a novel irrigating hood attached to the endoscope. Gastrointest Endosc 2003;57:732–5.

[68] Kume K, Yamasaki M, Yamasaki T, et al. Endoscopic hemostatic treatment under irrigation for upper-GI hemorrhage: a comparison of one third and total circumference transparent end hoods. Gastrointest Endosc 2004;59:712–6.

[69] Messmann H, Schaller P, Andus T, et al. Effect of programmed endoscopic follow-up examinations on the rebleeding rate of gastric or duodenal peptic ulcers treated by injection therapy: a prospective, randomized controlled trial. Endoscopy 1998;30:583–9.

[70] Villanueva C, Balanzo J, Torras X, et al. Value of second-look endoscopy after injection therapy for bleeding peptic ulcer: a prospective and randomized trial. Gastrointest Endosc 1994;40:34–9.

[71] Saeed ZA. Second thoughts about second-look endoscopy for ulcer bleeding? Endoscopy 1998;30:650–2.

[72] British Society of Gastroenterology Endoscopy Committee. Non-variceal upper gastrointestinal haemorrhage: guidelines. Gut 2002;51(Suppl 4):iv1–6.

[73] Lau JY, Sung JJ, Lam YH, et al. Endoscopic retreatment compared with surgery in patients with recurrent bleeding after initial endoscopic control of bleeding ulcers. N Engl J Med 1999;340:751–6.

[74] Wangensteen SL, Smith RB, Barker HG. Gastric cooling and gastric freezing. Surg Clin North Am 1966;46:463–75.

[75] Pasricha PJ, Hill S, Wadwa KS, et al. Endoscopic cryotherapy: experimental results and first clinical use. Gastrointest Endosc 1999;49:627–31.

[76] Kantsevoy SV, Cruz-Correa MR, Vaughn CA, et al. Endoscopic cryotherapy for the treatment of bleeding mucosal vascular lesions of the GI tract: a pilot study. Gastrointest Endosc 2003;57:403–6.

[77] Johnston CM, Schoenfeld LP, Mysore JV, et al. Endoscopic spray cryotherapy: a new technique for mucosal ablation in the esophagus. Gastrointest Endosc 1999;50:86–92.

[78] Walt RP, Cottrell J, Mann SG, et al. Continuous intravenous famotidine for haemorrhage from peptic ulcer. Lancet 1992;340:1058–62.

[79] Barer D, Ogilvie A, Henry D, et al. Cimetidine and tranexamic acid in the treatment of acute upper-gastrointestinal-tract bleeding. N Engl J Med 1983;308:1571–5.

[80] Collins R, Langman M. Treatment with histamine H2 antagonists in acute upper gastrointestinal hemorrhage. Implications of randomized trials. N Engl J Med 1985;313: 660–6.

[81] Selby NM, Kubba AK, Hawkey CJ. Acid suppression in peptic ulcer haemorrhage: a meta-analysis. Aliment Pharmacol Ther 2000;14:1119–26.

[82] Zed PJ, Loewen PS, Slavik RS, et al. Meta-analysis of proton pump inhibitors in treatment of bleeding peptic ulcers. Ann Pharmacother 2001;35:1528–34.

[83] Gisbert JP, Gonzalez L, Calvet X, et al. Proton pump inhibitors versus H2-antagonists: a meta-analysis of their efficacy in treating bleeding peptic ulcer. Aliment Pharmacol Ther 2001;15:917–26.

[84] Khuroo MS, Farahat KL, Kagevi IE. Treatment with proton pump inhibitors in acute non-variceal upper gastrointestinal bleeding: a meta-analysis. J Gastroenterol Hepatol 2005;20:11–25.

[85] Leontiadis GI, Sharma VK, Howden CW. Systematic review and meta-analysis of proton pump inhibitor therapy in peptic ulcer bleeding. BMJ 2005;330:568.

[86] Udd M, Miettinen P, Palmu A, et al. Regular-dose versus high-dose omeprazole in peptic ulcer bleeding: a prospective randomized double-blind study. Scand J Gastroenterol 2001;36:1332–8.

[87] Khuroo MS, Yattoo GN, Javid G, et al. A comparison of omeprazole and placebo for bleeding peptic ulcer. N Engl J Med 1997;336:1054–8.

[88] Kaviani MJ, Hashemi MR, Kazemifar AR, et al. Effect of oral omeprazole in reducing re-bleeding in bleeding peptic ulcers: a prospective, double-blind, randomized, clinical trial. Aliment Pharmacol Ther 2003;17:211–6.

[89] Javid G, Masoodi I, Zargar SA, et al. Omeprazole as adjuvant therapy to endoscopic combination injection sclerotherapy for treating bleeding peptic ulcer. Am J Med 2001;111: 280–4.

Gastroenterol Clin N Am 34 (2005) 623–642

GASTROENTEROLOGY CLINICS
OF NORTH AMERICA

Bleeding Caused by Portal Hypertension

Atif Zaman, MD, MPH[a], Naga Chalasani, MD[b],*

[a]Oregon Health Sciences University, 3181 Southwest Sam Jackson Park Road, PV 310, Portland, OR 97239, USA
[b]Indiana University School of Medicine, WD OPW 2005, 1001 West 10th Street, Indianapolis, IN 46202, USA

Variceal bleeding is one of the dreaded complications of portal hypertension. Although its prognosis has improved over the last several decades, it still carries substantial mortality. Although most portal hypertensive bleeds result from the ruptured distal esophageal varices, bleeding from other sources such gastric varices, portal hypertensive gastropathy, and ectopic varices can lead to clinically significant bleeding. The following sections review management of acute variceal bleeding, prevention of rebleeding, bleeding from gastric varices and portal hypertensive gastropathy, and the prevention of first variceal bleeding.

MANAGEMENT OF ACUTE VARICEAL BLEEDING

Variceal bleeding typically presents as massive gastrointestinal (GI) bleeding with hematemesis, melena, or hematochezia. In general, the therapeutic aims of management are to initially correct hypovolemia, to control bleeding, to prevent complications of bleeding, such as infection and renal failure, and to prevent early rebleeding.

INITIAL MANAGEMENT

Hemodynamic instability related to hypovolemia is a common presentation of acute variceal bleeding. Therefore, patients require prompt resuscitation, hemodynamic support, and correction of hemodynamic dysfunction, which usually requires intensive care unit monitoring. Lung aspiration of gastric contents and blood is a major concern, especially in encephalopathic patients. Furthermore, patients who are actively consuming alcohol can be combative and difficult to sedate for endoscopic procedures. Therefore, endotracheal intubation for airway protection should be considered in anyone who is at risk for aspiration or is uncooperative. Judicious transfusion of blood products is necessary.

*Corresponding author. E-mail address: nchalasa@iupui.edu (N. Chalasani).

0889-8553/05/$ – see front matter
doi:10.1016/j.gtc.2005.08.008

In animal studies, 100% volume replacement in portal hypertensive rats led to a rebound increase in portal pressure [1]. In another study, following a variceal bleed in animal models, rapid blood transfusion to correct arterial pressure led to an increased risk of further bleeding [2]. Therefore, one should aim for target hemoglobin between 9 and 10 g/dL when transfusing cirrhotic patients who have variceal bleeding.

Renal failure is a common complication of cirrhotic patients hospitalized for variceal bleeding [3]. The cause of acute renal failure in this setting is typically multifactorial, including prolonged hypovolemia, overuse of diuretics, infection, and hepatorenal syndrome. In a retrospective study by Cardenas and colleagues [3], hypovolemia and poor liver function were the only independent risk factors for renal failure in patients who had cirrhosis presenting with upper GI hemorrhage. Furthermore, in this study, renal failure was an independent risk factor for in-hospital mortality. Therefore, every effort should be made to avoid the development of renal failure by early aggressive resuscitation of patients and by avoiding nephrotoxic agents such as aminoglycosides and nonsteroidal drugs.

Recent studies have shown the importance of using prophylactic antibiotics in cirrhotic patients with bleeding. Bacterial infections are more common in cirrhotic patients with variceal bleeding (35% to 66%) than in noncirrhotic hospitalized patients (5% to 7%) [4]. Two factors have been identified to increase the risk of bacterial infections in patients who have cirrhosis: severity of the liver disease and GI hemorrhage [5,6]. Several studies have shown that mortality is significantly higher in infected cirrhotic patients versus noninfected cirrhotic patients [7,8]. Furthermore, a study by Bernard and colleagues demonstrated that infected cirrhotic patients had a higher rate of variceal rebleeding (43%, 10 of 23 patients) than noninfected patients (10%, 4 of 41 patients) [9]. This is likely because of the endotoxins and cytokines as a consequence of the infection, which induces hematologic abnormalities, including platelet dysfunction and activation of coagulation and fibrinolytic systems [10]. Therefore, the current body of knowledge strongly suggests that, in patients who have cirrhosis with variceal hemorrhage, prophylaxis against a bacterial infection reduces variceal rebleeding and improves survival. A meta-analysis by Bernard and colleagues [11] demonstrated that prophylactic use of antibiotics significantly increased survival (9.1% mean improvement, $P = .004$). A recent randomized study by Hou and colleagues [12] showed that early rebleeding (within the first 15 days) was significantly lower in patients who received ofloxacin for 7 days compared with those who received on-demand antibiotics (8% versus 38%, $P < .05$). In prospective studies, the most common causes of bacterial infections in patients who had cirrhosis with variceal bleeding included spontaneous bacterial peritonitis, urinary tract infection, and pneumonia. Typically gram-negative organisms are isolated [6,13]. Therefore, antibiotics (oral quinolones or intravenous cephalosporins) should be given for 7 days in patients who have cirrhosis with bleeding.

As a part of the initial stabilization, balloon tamponade with a Sengtaken-Blakemore tube may be necessary to control brisk bleeding. Balloon tamponade successfully achieves hemostasis in 90% of cases of bleeding varices, but it has a high recurrence rate for rebleeding once the balloon is deflated. Therefore, balloon tamponade should be reserved as a rescue procedure, so that patients are stabilized for a more definitive therapy.

MANAGEMENT OF BLEEDING

Vasoactive Agents

Vasoactive agents for treating bleeding esophageal varices first were described in 1962. Vasopressin was the first agent studied [14] because of its ability to induce splanchnic vasoconstriction, which leads to a decrease in portal inflow and portal pressure. A meta-analysis by D'Amico and colleagues of 157 patients demonstrated a significant reduction in failure to control bleeding from 82% to 50%, with no difference in mortality [15]. Vasopressin, however, leads to systemic vasoconstriction in addition to splanchnic vasoconstriction. Vasopressin's cardiovascular adverse effects, such as myocardial ischemia and infarction, has limited is use. Combining glyceril-trinitrate with vasopressin has reduced adverse effects and improved efficacy over vasopressin alone [16,17]. Because of the significant adverse effects of vasopressin-based therapy, future research has been aimed at developing more effective and safer agents.

Somatostatin is a natural peptide that induces splanchnic vasoconstriction, which leads to a decrease in portal pressure. It lacks most of the cardiovascular adverse effects seen with vasopressin. In four unblinded randomized studies, compared with placebo, somatostatin showed a trend toward benefit, with an overall risk reduction by 17% [18]. One study by Avgerinos and colleagues [19] observed that somatostatin given before urgent sclerotherapy made the endoscopic procedure easier in the acute setting. None of these studies, however, demonstrated an improvement in overall survival compared with placebo. When compared with vasopressin [18], somatostatin was equivalent in terms of efficacy in controlling bleeding but had significantly fewer adverse effects. When somatostatin was compared with emergency sclerotherapy in 367 patients from four randomized controlled trials [20–23], there was no difference between the two groups in terms of failure to control bleeding, rebleeding, and mortality. On the other hand, the somatostatin group had fewer complications. A study by Villaneuva and colleagues [24], however, compared somatostatin alone (n = 50) with combined therapy of somatostatin and sclerotherapy (n = 50). This study observed a higher rate of therapeutic failure in the somatostatin alone group in terms of failure to control bleeding, transfusion requirements, and rebleeding. Therefore, the data suggest that the greatest benefit of somatostatin is when it is used in conjunction with endoscopic therapy. Unfortunately, somatostatin is not available in the United States.

Octreotide, a somatostatin analog, is available in the United States. It has similar properties as somatostatin, but with a longer biological half-life. Results regarding its efficacy compared with placebo, sclerotherapy, and balloon tamponade have been inconsistent. Many of the studies were small, low quality, and unblinded. A recent meta-analysis [25] demonstrated that octreotide was superior to other alternative therapies (placebo, vasopressin/terlipressin, or sclerotherapy) in controlling acute variceal bleeding (relative risk 0.63; 95% confidence interval [CI] 0.51 to 0.77). Because of its excellent safety profile, octreotide has an added benefit that it can be administered in outside of the intensive care unit setting.

Terlipressin is a long acting triglycyl-lysine derivative of vasopressin. It is transformed slowly to vasopressin by enzymatic cleavage. Because of this slow release to the active agent, terlipressin has significantly fewer adverse effects than vasopressin. Also, because of its long half-life, terlipressin can be administered at home or the emergency room with significant reduction in failure to control bleeding [26]. Furthermore, in a study by Brunati and colleagues [27] comparing terlipressin with terlipressin plus sclerotherapy, the combination group had significantly better control of active bleeding and less transfusion requirements. Currently terlipressin is the only pharmacologic therapy that has been shown to reduce mortality in acute variceal hemorrhage compared with placebo (relative risk 0.66, 95% CI 0.49 to 0.88) [28]. Unfortunately, terlipressin is not available in the United States.

There has been recent interest in the use of recombinant factor VIIa (rFVIIa) for managing upper GI hemorrhage in patients with cirrhosis. Cirrhotic patients often will have defects in the coagulation system, in particular factor VII deficiency. Bosch and colleagues [29] performed a randomized control trial of 245 cirrhotic patients presenting with upper GI hemorrhage to evaluate if the addition of rFVIIa to standard therapy improves control of bleeding. Patients either received 8 doses of 100 µg/kg of rFVIIa or placebo. Recombinant factor VIIa did not show advantage over standard therapy in the whole study population. In patients who had decompensated cirrhosis (Child-Pugh class C), however, better 24-hour bleeding control was achieved in the rFVIIa group ($P = .01$). These findings need to be validated further. In addition, questions such as the optimal dose of rFVIIa and its use as first-line or salvage therapy need to be answered before its routine use can be recommended in this setting.

Endoscopic Management

Both sclerotherapy and band ligation are very effective in controlling acute esophageal variceal bleeding and preventing rebleeding during the index hospitalization. These two modalities are the mainstay of therapy, and they are successful in achieving hemostasis in 80% to 90% of patients with acute variceal bleeding. The advantages of sclerotherapy include its ease of use, especially during massive bleeding, and its lower cost. Sclerotherapy, however, has been associated with ulceration and bleeding, bacteremia, and stricture formation. Band ligation has a lower rate of complication, but it can be difficult to use during acute bleeding. Studies have shown that the two modalities are comparable in achieving initial hemostasis [30]. A more recent study by Avgerinos and colleagues [31] demonstrated that after initial control of bleeding, band ligation had significantly fewer rebleeding rates and complications, and it achieved eradication with fewer endoscopic sessions than sclerotherapy. Therefore, wherever feasible, band ligation should be the first-line endoscopic therapy for acute variceal bleeding. There are some data regarding the use of endoscopically delivered tissue adhesives, such as cyanoacrylate, for treating esophageal variceal bleeding. A study by Feretis and colleagues [32] observed that cyanoacrylate in combination with polidocanol did not control active bleeding significantly better than polidocanol alone (95% versus 78%). Recurrent bleeding over 2 month, however, was significantly less in the combination group. Sung and colleagues [33] demonstrated that cyanoacrylate was similar to endoscopic band ligation in achieving initial control of bleeding (100% in each group), but cyanoacrylate was inferior to banding for preventing rebleeding over a 7- to 8-month follow up (67% vs. 28%). Because of the sparse data available regarding the use of tissue adhesives for managing bleeding caused by esophageal varices and the inherent difficulties in using these compounds, their use cannot be recommended. In addition, these agents are not approved for use in the United States for managing varices. As mentioned in the previous section, the use of vasoactive agents in combination with endoscopic therapy appears to be more efficacious than either therapy alone.

Transjugular Intrahepatic Portosystemic Shunt

Transjugular intrahepatic portosystemic shunt (TIPS) is indicated in situations when acutely bleeding varices are refractory to medical therapy. TIPS has been shown in this situation to control bleeding in 95% of cases with a rebleed rate of only 18% [34]. Furthermore, a study by Vangeli and colleagues [35] reviewed 15 studies involving the use of TIPS to control bleeding when medical therapy failed. Similar to previous reports, bleeding was controlled in 93.6% of patients, and rebled within 7 days was low (12.4%). The mortality rate, however, is between 30% and 40%. This is likely because patients with continued bleeding tend to be quite ill and have a high mortality rate despite any intervention.

Surgery

Surgical options include selective portosystemic shunting, calibrated H grafts, and devascularization procedures. The 30-day mortality rate, however, approaches 80% with these procedures [36]. Therefore, in most situations, surgical intervention for acute variceal bleeding should be reserved for when medical therapy fails and TIPS is not available.

Fig. 1 outlines a reasonable algorithm for the management of acute variceal hemorrhage.

PREVENTING RECURRENT VARICEAL BLEEDING

Without further therapy, once initial control of is achieved, variceal bleeding recurs in two thirds of patients within 2 months [37]. Factors associated with increase risk of recurrent bleeding include presence of active bleeding on initial endoscopy, large varices, severity of initial hemorrhage, degree of hepatic

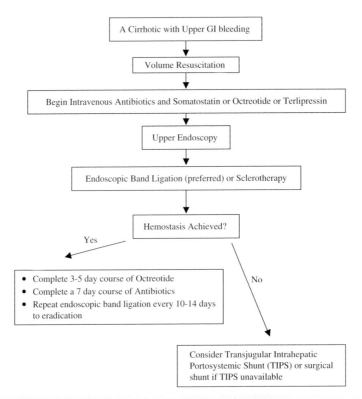

Fig. 1. Suggested algorithm for managing acute variceal bleeding.

decompensation, impaired renal function, presence of encephalopathy, and severe portal hypertension (as measured by the hepatic venous pressure gradient) [38]. Because of the high risk of recurrent hemorrhage, secondary prophylaxis should be initiated shortly after an episode of bleeding.

Pharmacologic Therapy

The main goal of pharmacologic is to significantly reduce portal hypertension, ideally to reduce the hepatic venous pressure gradient below12 mmHg, and to prevent recurrent bleeding. Therefore, the ideal way to adjust medical therapy would be to follow portal pressure as determined by the hepatic venous pressure gradient. The best time to measure portal pressure would be within the first month after a bleeding episode to determine which patients have severe portal hypertension and have the greatest risk of recurrent bleeding. More than a 20% reduction in portal pressure has been shown to significantly reduce the cumulative probability of recurrent bleeding from 28% to 4% in the first year and from 39% to 9% at 2 years [39]. Unfortunately, pressure measurements are expensive, invasive, and not readily available. Therefore, surrogate measures of portal pressure reduction commonly are used, such as a target heart rate of 55 beats per minute or a 25% reduction in the heart rate from base-line. Not all patients, however, are protected from bleeding. Recent studies have shown that despite adequate beta-blocker therapy, there are a percentage of patients that still have hepatic venous pressure gradients above 12 mmHg, which puts them at continued risk for variceal hemorrhage [40].

Several trials have demonstrated the efficacy of a nonselective beta-blocker compared with placebo in decreasing the risk of recurrent bleeding and improving survival [41]. The addition of isorbide mononitrate (ISMN) to a beta-blocker regimen appears to further reduce the rate of rebleeding [42]. In addition, recent studies have shown that combination pharmacologic therapy may be superior to sclerotherapy and band ligation. Incidence of rebleeding was 25% over an 18-month period with combination medical therapy compared with 53% for sclerotherapy in Child-Pugh class A or B cirrhotics [43]. These same investigators compared combination therapy with band ligation and demonstrated a reduction in bleeding frequency from 49% to 33% [44]. The benefit of combined medical therapy, however, was realized mainly in patients who had Child-Pugh class A or B cirrhosis. More recent studies comparing combination pharmacologic therapy with band ligation revealed conflicting results. Lo and colleagues [45] observed that band ligation was superior to combination medical therapy. A study by Patch and colleagues [46] observed that both treatment modalities were equivalent. Most likely the differences in results lie in study methods. Combination therapy may be superior to endoscopic therapy. The adverse effects of pharmacologic therapy, especially with combination pharmacologic medical therapy, however, can limit compliance.

Endoscopic therapy

Even though sclerotherapy has been shown to be effective in reducing recurrent variceal hemorrhage and appears to be equivalent to beta-blocker therapy [47], band ligation appears to have similar efficacy in decreasing recurrent bleeding, but fewer complications and higher survival rates [48]. Therefore, for endoscopic therapy to prevent rebleeding, band ligation should be considered the procedure of choice. Combination band ligation with pharmacologic therapy may be the ideal treatment modality. So far, there have been two published trials comparing band ligation alone with band ligation plus pharmacologic therapy. In a study by Lo and colleagues comparing band ligation alone with band ligation plus nadolol and sucralfate, rebleeding was reduced from 47% to 23% with combination therapy [49]. A more recent study by Pena and colleagues comparing band ligation alone with band ligation plus nadolol, demonstrated that the rebleeding rate was reduced from 38% to 14% with the combination group [50]. In addition, postbanding ulcers are common, and significant bleeding from these ulcers occurs in 2% to 5% of cases. Varices rebleeding rates potentially can be reduced further by adding antiulcer therapy after endoscopic therapy. Shaheen and colleagues [51] performed a study to evaluate the efficacy of proton pump inhibitor in treating postbanding ulcers in the setting of elective endoscopic band ligation. This was a randomized, double-blinded, placebo-controlled trial. After elective endoscopic band ligation, subjects received either intravenous pantoprazole 40 mg followed by 40 mg oral pantoprazole daily for 9 days (n = 22) or intravenous/oral placebo (n = 22). There was no difference in the number of postbanding ulcers among the groups. Ulcers in the control group, however, were twice as large as the pantoprazole group (82 mm^2 versus 37 mm^2, $P < .01$). Two patients had postbanding ulcer bleeding; both were in the control group ($P > .05$). Because proton pump inhibitors are tolerated well and simple to administer, their use in this setting appears reasonable.

Surgical Shunt and Transjugular Intrahepatic Portosystemic Shunt Procedures

Portocaval or distal splenorenal shunts have been used in preventing recurrent variceal bleeding. A meta-analysis comparing distal splenorenal shunt with sclerotherapy found that shunt placement significantly reduced the rate of recurrent bleeding but also increased the incidence of encephalopathy and did not improve survival [52]. Rebleeding after surgical shunts typically is caused by shunt thrombosis, which occurs usually within the first year. It is unusual for surgical shunts to thrombose beyond 1 year. Similarly, with TIPS compared with endoscopic therapy the rebleeding rate was significantly lower with TIPS, 19% versus 47%, but the incidence of encephalopathy was higher with TIPS, 34% versus 19%, with no difference in survival [53]. Rosemurgy and colleagues compared TIPS with a surgically place H-graft shunt. This was a nonrandomized study of 132 patients. Rosemurgy and colleagues observed that the frequency of rebleeding was significantly less in the surgical group (3% versus 16%), and the patients who had TIPS required frequent interventions to maintain shunt patency. Thirty-day mortality rates, however, were higher in the surgical group, 43% versus 15% [54]. Therefore, surgical shunts should be used to prevent rebleeding in patients who do not tolerate or are not compliant with medical therapy and have relatively preserved liver function. TIPS should be reserved for patients who have poor liver function and who have failed medical therapy. Fig. 2 outlines a reasonable algorithm for preventing recurrent variceal hemorrhage.

BLEEDING FROM PORTAL HYPERTENSIVE GASTROPATHY

Portal hypertensive gastropathy (PHG) is the characteristic mosaic-like gastric mucosa with or without red spots; it is seen quite frequently in patients with both cirrhotic as well as noncirrhotic portal hypertension [55]. The histology of PHG is quite typical, and it reveals dilated capillaries and venules in the mucosa and submucosa without erosion, inflammation, or fibrin thrombi [56]. Although there are several published methods for grading portal gastropathy, the classification proposed by McCormack and colleagues appears to be the most widely used and reproducible [56]. According to this grading, PHG is classified into mild (fine pink speckles, superficial reddening, or mucosal mosaic pattern) or severe (discrete red spots or diffuse hemorrhagic lesions) categories

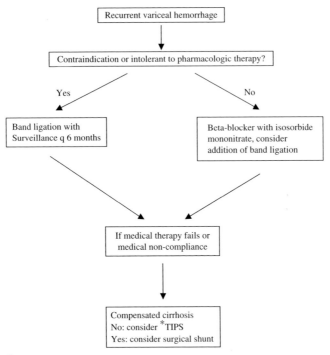

Fig. 2. Suggested algorithm for preventing recurrent variceal hemorrhage.

[56] (Fig. 3). Although the bleeding from PHG can be acute or chronic in nature, chronic bleeding presenting as iron deficiency anemia or occult blood in stool is far more frequent than acute bleeding [57–59]. In three recently published papers, the incidence of hemodynamically significant acute bleeding from PHG was less than 5% [57–59]. The specific treatment options for significant PHG include nonselective beta-blockers, endoscopic therapy, or TIPS or surgical shunts [55]. Nonselective beta-blockers have been shown to reduce the risk of bleeding in patients who have PHG [60–62]. In one study, compared with placebo, propranolol significantly reduced the risk of bleeding in patients who had severe PHG at 12 months (35% versus 62%) and 30 months (48% versus 93%) [62]. Endoscopic therapy in the form of cauterization (heater or bipolar probe or argon plasma coagulation) or injection sclerotherapy can be effective in patients who have acute bleeding caused by PHG. The role of endoscopic therapy for managing clinically significant chronic bleeding, however, is less clear. For these patients, it is not unreasonable to attempt endoscopic therapy with argon plasma coagulation, especially if such endoscopic expertise is available locally. TIPS can reduce the bleeding from severe PHG effectively, but it should be reserved for patients who are transfusion-dependent despite maximal medical and endoscopic therapy [63,64].

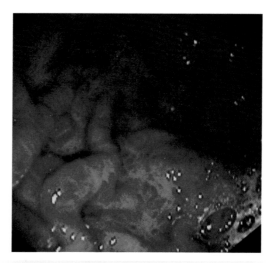

Fig. 3. Severe portal hypertensive gastropathy. Gastric body and antrum reveal discrete red spots intermingled with diffuse hemorrhagic lesions.

Sometimes, patients who have portal hypertension present with bleeding from mucosal lesions resembling gastric antral vascular ectasia (GAVE) or watermelon stomach [59]. Although the pathogenesis of GAVE is not related to portal hypertension, its prevalence appears to be higher in patients who have cirrhosis and portal hypertension [59]. Although it usually is offered, the effectiveness of endoscopic laser therapy in portal hypertensive patients with GAVE is unclear. TIPS plays no significant role in the management of GAVE in patients who have cirrhosis and portal hypertension [63].

BLEEDING FROM GASTRIC VARICES

Gastric varices are rare but important sources for bleeding in patients who have portal hypertension [65–67]. Gastric varices can be classified into gastro–esophageal varices (GOV) or isolated gastric varices (IGV) [68]. GOV are classified further into GOV 1 (in continuity with esophageal varices and extend 2 to 5 cm below the gastroesophageal junction) or GOV 2 (esophageal varices extending into the fundus). IGV can be located in the fundus (IGV 1) or body/antrum (IGV 2) (Fig. 4). Gastric varices located in the gastric fundus (either GOV 2 or IGV 1) carry a greater risk of bleeding than those located in other parts of the stomach [68].

Potential treatments for gastric variceal bleeding include endoscopic (cyanoacrylate or its derivatives or thrombin), radiological (TIPS or balloon-occluded retrograde transvenous obliteration), and surgical (gastric devascularization and splenectomy, surgical shunts, or liver transplantation) modalities [69–78].

Endoscopic therapy with N-butyl-2-cyanoacrylate (cyanoacrylate) is very effective in providing acute hemostasis and in reducing rebleeding in patients

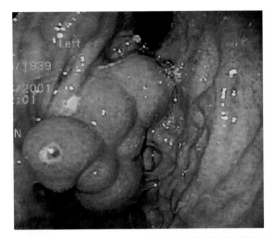

Fig. 4. Isolated large gastric varices in the gastric fundus (IGV1) with high-risk stigmata. Gastric varices of this type carry high risk of bleeding and thus should be provided primary prophylaxis.

who have bleeding gastric varices [69–72]. Peripheral embolization (to lungs, brain, or viscera) is a rare but important complication of cyanoacrylate therapy. Although this form of therapy is used widely in Europe and Asia, cyanoacrylate is not commercially available and seldom is used in the United States [69].

Studies have shown that TIPS is effective in providing acute hemostasis and in reducing rebleeding in patients with gastric variceal bleeding [73,74]. In some patients, however, TIPS may not be effective because of insufficient anterograde portal venous blood flow caused by extensive collaterals. In these patients, selective embolization of the collaterals may improve the effectiveness of TIPS by enhancing the anterograde flow.

Balloon-occluded retrograde transvenous obliteration (B-RTO) is a newly developed technique performed by the interventional radiologists to treat gastric fundal varices associated with spontaneous gastro–renal shunts [75]. This procedure employs ethanolamine oleate to obliterate fundal varices, feeding vessels and the gastro–renal shunt. Several Japanese studies have shown that this form of therapy is effective in selected patients with gastric variceal bleeding who also have gastro–renal shunts [75,76]. More recently, Shiba and colleagues reported that balloon-occluded injection sclerotherapy is safe and effective for treating high-risk gastric varices; the procedure can be performed even in patients without gastro–renal shunts [79].

As there are relatively few randomized controlled trials investigating the relative efficacy of various treatment modalities, the management of gastric variceal bleeding is controversial and geographically variable. At most institutions in the United States, TIPS usually is considered as the first line of therapy for patients with gastric variceal bleeding.

Although some studies have advocated prophylactic endoscopic therapy for high-risk gastric varices [79,80], primary prophylaxis against gastric variceal bleeding has not been investigated adequately. Until more data become available showing the safety and efficacy of prophylactic endoscopic therapy, it is the authors' opinion that patients with high-risk gastric varices who have never bled before should be treated with maximal doses of nonselective beta-blockers.

PREVENTING THE FIRST VARICEAL BLEEDING (PRIMARY PROPHYLAXIS)

As each episode of variceal bleeding carries significant risk of morbidity and mortality, it is essential that primary prophylaxis should be considered in every patient who has suspected or proven cirrhosis. It has been recommended that all patients with cirrhosis (either suspected or diagnosed) should undergo diagnostic upper endoscopy. those who are found to have high-risk gastro–esophageal varices should receive treatment to prevent the first variceal bleed [81–83]. Patients who have large gastro–esophageal varices (irrespective of Child-Pugh score or presence of red signs) and those with small varices bearing red signs are at risk for rupture and thus should be offered prophylactic therapy (Fig. 5).

Recent studies have identified that certain nonendoscopic variables can predict the presence of varices (or large varices). These variables include thrombocytopenia, splenomegaly, portal vein diameter by ultrasonography, or Child's C cirrhosis [84]. Based on the presence or absence of these variables, some investigators have developed models to predict the presence of varices or large varices [85]. These models are promising but lack optimal precision. Until validated prediction models with clinically acceptable precision are available, endoscopic screening is the best practice to detect and risk stratify gastro–esophageal varices [83].

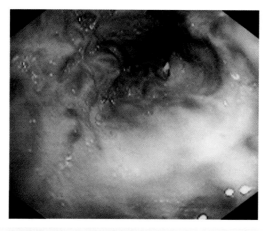

Fig. 5. Large esophageal varices in the distal esophagus.

Therapeutic options for primary prophylaxis include nonselective beta-blockers and prophylactic endoscopic banding (Fig. 6). Nonselective beta-blockers (propranolol or Nadolol) significantly reduce the risk of first variceal bleeding and remain the treatment of choice for patients with high-risk varices [85]. When beta-blockers are given for the primary prophylaxis, the dosage should be titrated to a heart rate of 55 beats per minute. Many patients, however, may not tolerate beta-blockers because of adverse effects (asthenia, sexual dysfunction, or hypotension) requiring their discontinuation [85]. The monitoring of hepatic venous pressure gradient can identify precisely those who will benefit the most from pharmacotherapy. Its utility, however, has not been tested in clinical trials [86,87]. If nonselective beta-blockers are provided for primary prophylaxis, their administration should be continued indefinitely, as their discontinuation can lead to significantly increased risk of bleeding [88]. Studies have shown that isosorbide mononitrate as monotherapy is not effective in preventing the first variceal bleed, and thus it should not be used for primary prophylaxis [83].

The role of endoscopic ligation as a primary prophylactic measure has been investigated in the recent years. In comparison to no therapy, in patients with moderate-to-large esophageal varices, prophylactic endoscopic banding leads to a significant reduction in the incidence of first variceal bleeding and improves survival [89] (Table 1). Prophylactic banding has been compared with nonselective beta-blockers in several randomized controlled studies, and two meta-analyses that aggregated the results of these studies were published [89,90] (Table 2). Prophylactic banding is more effective than beta-blockers in preventing the first variceal bleeding in patients with moderate-to-large esophageal varices,

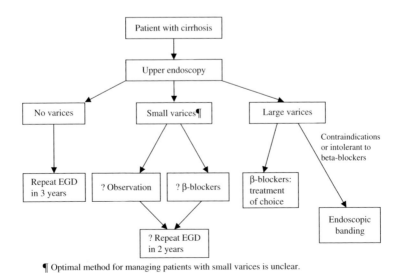

¶ Optimal method for managing patients with small varices is unclear.

Fig. 6. Suggested algorithm for preventing first variceal bleeding.

Table 1
Meta-analysis of studies that compared endoscopic ligation to no prophylactic treatment (601 subjects in five randomized studies)

Outcomes	Relative risk (CI)	Relative risk reduction	NNT (CI)
First esophageal variceal bleed	0.36 (0.26–0.50)	64%	4 (3–6)
Bleed-related mortality	0.20 (0.11–0.39)	80%	7 (5–11)
All-cause mortality	0.55 (0.43–0.71)	45%	5 (4–9)

Modified from Imperiale TF, Chalasani N. A meta-analysis of endoscopic variceal ligation in primary prophylaxis of esophageal variceal bleeding in patients with cirrhosis. Hepatology 2001;33:821–5; with permission.

but it offers no survival advantage over nonselective beta-blockers [82,89,90] (Table 2). The long-term benefits of prophylactic banding are unclear, as most studies had modest duration of follow-up. Furthermore, the effects of prophylactic banding as compared with beta-blockers on the cost-effectiveness and quality of life have not been addressed adequately. Until more studies addressing these issues are available, prophylactic endoscopic banding should be offered to patients with moderate-to-large varices who are intolerant to or have contraindications for nonselective beta-blocker therapy [82].

Two recent studies have evaluated if nonselective beta-blockers can modify the natural history of portal hypertension in patients with small varices or no portal hypertension [91,92]. In one study, 161 cirrhotic patients who with small esophageal varices who have never bled before were randomized to receive nadolol (n = 83) or placebo (n = 78) and were followed for a mean duration of 36 months [91]. Compared with placebo, patients receiving nadolol had significantly lower development of large varices and lower incidence of bleeding [91]. In another multi-center study, 213 patients who had cirrhosis with portal hypertension (defined as hepatic vein pressure gradient greater than 5 mmHG) but no esophageal varices were randomized to receive timolol or placebo [92]. In this study, timolol therapy had no effect on the development of varices, variceal hemorrhage, ascites, or death. The findings of these two studies suggest

Table 2
Meta-analysis of studies that compared ligation with propranolol (481 patients in five clinical trials)

Outcome	Relative risk (95% CI)	NNT
First esophageal variceal bleed	0.56 (0.36–0.87)	10
Bleed-related mortality	0.84 (0.44–1.61)	-
All-cause mortality	1.03 (0.78–1.36)	-
Severe adverse events	0.36 (0.16–0.72)	9

Modified from Khuroo MS, et al. Meta-analysis: endoscopic variceal ligation for primary prophylaxis of oesophageal variceal bleeding. Aliment Pharmacol Ther 2005;21:347–61; with permission.

that primary prophylaxis with nonselective beta blockers can be provided to cirrhotics with small esophageal varices but not to those with no varices [91,92].

Several cost-effectiveness analyses have found that a strategy of universal beta-blocker therapy to all cirrhotics without subjecting them to upper endoscopy is more cost-effective than other strategies of providing primary prophylaxis [93–95]. The only clinical trial that tested the strategy of universal beta-blocker therapy, however, did not find it to be effective [96]. Until more data become available, the authors do not recommend the strategy of universal beta-blockers (without investigating their varices status), as it would subject a large number of cirrhotics without gastroesophageal varices (approximately 50%) to an indefinite therapy with unpleasant adverse effects. Indeed, the recently concluded Baveno IV consensus workshop recommended that it is not indicated to treat patients who have cirrhosis with beta-blockers without prior assessment of the presence of esophageal varices [83].

SUMMARY

Variceal bleeding is one of the dreaded complications of portal hypertension. Patients who have suspected or proven cirrhosis should undergo diagnostic upper endoscopy to detect medium and large gastro–esophageal varices. Patients with medium and large gastro–esophageal varices should be treated with nonselective beta-blockers (propranolol or nadolol), and these agents should be titrated to a heart rate of 55 beats per minute or adverse effects. If there are contraindications to or if patients are intolerant to beta-blockers, it is appropriate to consider prophylactic banding therapy for individuals with medium-to-large esophageal varices. When patients who have cirrhosis present with GI bleeding, they should be resuscitated and receive octreotide or other vasoactive agents. Endoscopy should be performed promptly to diagnose the source of bleeding and to provide endoscopic therapy (preferably banding). The currently available treatment for acute variceal bleeding provides hemostasis in most patients. These patients, however, are at significant risk for rebleeding unless secondary prophylaxis is provided. Although various pharmacological, endoscopic, radiological, and surgical options are available, combined pharmacological and endoscopic therapy is the most common form of secondary prophylaxis. TIPS is a radiologically placed portasystemic shunt, and if placed in suitable patients, it can provide effective treatment for patients with variceal bleeding that is refractory to medical and endoscopic therapy.

References

[1] Kravetz D, Bosch J, Arderiu M, et al. Abnormalities in organ blood flow and its distribution during expiratory pressure ventilation. Hepatology 1989;9:808–14.

[2] Castaneda B, Morales J, Lionetti R, et al. Effects of blood volume reinstitution following a portal hypertensive-related bleeding in anesthetized cirrhotic rats. Hepatology 2001;33: 821–5.

[3] Cardenas A, Gines P, Uriz J, et al. Renal failure after upper gastrointestinal bleeding in cirrhosis: Incidence, clinical course, predictive factors, and short term prognosis. Hepatology 2001;34:671–6.

[4] Goulis J, Patch D, Burroughs AK. Bacterial infection in the pathogenesis of variceal hemorrhage. Lancet 1999;353(9147):139–42.
[5] Pauwels A, Mostefa-Kara N, Debenes B, et al. Systemic antibiotic prophylaxis after gastrointestinal hemorrhage in cirrhotic patients with a high risk of infection. Hepatology 1996;24:802–6.
[6] Blaise M, Pateron D, Trinchet C, et al. Systemic antibiotic therapy prevents bacterial infection in cirrhotic patients with gastrointestinal hemorrhage. Hepatology 1994;20:34–8.
[7] Bleichner G, Boulanger R, Squara P, et al. Frequency of infections in cirrhotic patients presenting with acute gastrointestinal hemorrhage. Br J Surg 1986;73:724–6.
[8] Caly WR, Strauss E. A prospective study of bacterial infections in patients with cirrhosis. J Hepatol 1993;18:353–8.
[9] Bernard B, Cadranell JF, Valla D, et al. Prognostic significance of bacterial infection in bleeding cirrhotic patients: a prospective study. Gastroenterology 1995;108:1828–34.
[10] Papatheodoridis GV, Patch D, Webster JM, et al. Infection and hemostasis in decompensated cirrhosis: a prospective study using thromboelastography. Hepatology 1999;29:1085–90.
[11] Bernard B, Nguyen KE, Opolon P, et al. Antibiotic prophylaxis (ABP) for the prevention of bacterial infections in cirrhotic patients with gastrointestinal bleeding (GB): a meta-analysis. Hepatology 1999;29:1655–61.
[12] Hou MC, Lin HC, Liu TT, et al. Antibiotic prophylaxis after endoscopic therapy prevents rebleeding in acute variceal hemorrhage: a randomized trial. Hepatology 2004;39(3):746–53.
[13] Rimola A, Bory F, Teres J, et al. Oral, nonabsorbable antibiotics prevent infection in cirrhotics with gastrointestinal hemorrhage. Hepatology 1985;5:463–7.
[14] Merigan TC, Plotkin GR, Davidson CS. Effect of intravenously administered posterior pituitary extract on hemorrhage from bleeding esophageal varices. N Engl J Med 1962;266:134–5.
[15] D'Amico G, Pagliaro L, Bosch J. The treatment of hypertension: A meta-analytic review. Hepatology 1995;22:332–54.
[16] Tsai YT, Lay CS, Lai KH, et al. Controlled trial of vasopressin plus nitroglycerin vs vasopressin alone in the treatment of bleeding oesophageal varices. Hepatology 1986;6:406–9.
[17] Bosch J, Groszmann RJ, Garcia-Pagan JC, et al. Association of transdermal nitroglycerin to vasopressin infusion in the treatment of variceal haemorrhage: a placebo-controlled clinical trial. Hepatology 1989;10:962–8.
[18] D'Amico G, Pagliaro L, Bosch J. Pharmacologic treatment of portal hypertension: An evidenced approach. Semin Liver Dis 1999;19:475–505.
[19] Avgerinos A, Nevens F, Raptis S, et al. Early administration of somatostatin and efficacy of sclerotherapy in acute variceal bleeds: the European Acute Bleeding Oesophageal Variceal Episodes (ABOVE) randomised trial. Lancet 1997;350:1495–9.
[20] DiFebo G, Siringo S, Vacirca M, et al. Somatostatin and urgent sclerotherapy in active esophageal variceal bleeding. Gastroenterolgy 1990;98:A583.
[21] Shields R, Jenkins SA, Baxter JN, et al. A prospective randomized controlled trial comparing the efficacy of somatostatin with injection sclerotherapy in the control of oesophageal varices. J Hepatol 1992;16:128–37.
[22] Planas R, Quer JC, Boix J, et al. A prospective randomized trial comparing somatostatin and sclerotherapy in the treatment of acute variceal bleeding. Hepatology 1994;20:370–5.
[23] Escorsell A, Bordas JM, Ruiz del Arbol L, et al. Randomized control trial of sclerotherapy versus somatostatin infusion in the prevention of early rebleeding following acute variceal hemorrhage in patients with cirrhosis. J Hepatol 1998;29:779–88.
[24] Villanueva C, Ortiz J, Sabat M, et al. Somatostatin alone or combined with emergency sclerotherapy in the treatment of acute esophageal variceal bleeding: a prospective randomized trial. Hepatology 1999;30:384–9.

[25] Corley DA, Cello JP, Adkisson W, et al. Octreotide for acute esophageal variceal bleeding: Meta-analysis. Gastroenterology 2001;120:946–54.

[26] Levacher S, Letoumalin P, Pateron D, et al. Early administration of terlipressin plus glyceryl trinitrate to control active upper gastrointestinal bleeding in cirrhotic patients. Lancet 1995;346:865–8.

[27] Brunati S, Ceriani R, Curioni R, et al. Sclerotherapy alone vs. sclerotherapy plus sclerotherapy plus octreotide in the treatment of acute variceal haemorrhage. Hepatology 1996;24:A207.

[28] Ioannu GN, Doust J, Rockey D. Systematic review: Terlipressin in acute oesophageal variceal hemorrhage. Aliment Pharmacol Ther 2003;17:53–64.

[29] Bosch J, Thiabut D, Bendtsen F, et al. Recombinant factor VIIa for upper gastrointestinal bleeding in patients with cirrhosis: a randomized, double-blind trial. Gastroenterology 2004;127:1123–30.

[30] Steigmann GV, Goff JS, Michaletz-Onody P, et al. Endoscopic sclerotherapy as compared with endoscopic ligation for bleeding esophageal varices. N Engl J Med 1992;326:1527–32.

[31] Avgerinos A, Armonis A, Manolakpoulos S, et al. Endoscopic sclerotherapy versus variceal ligation in the long-term management of patients with cirrhosis after variceal bleeding: a prospective randomized study. J Hepatol 1997;26:1034–41.

[32] Feretis C, Dimopoulos C, Benakis P, et al. N-butyl-2-cyanoacrylate (Histoacryl) plus sclerotherapy versus sclerotherapy alone in the treatment of bleeding esophageal varices: a randomized prospective study. Endoscopy 1995;27:355–7.

[33] Sung JY, Lee TY, Suen R, et al. Banding is superior to cyanoacrylate for the treatment of esophageal variceal bleeding: a prospective randomized trial. Gastrointest Endosc 1998;47:A77.

[34] Burroughs AK, Patch D. Transjugular intrahepatic portosystemic shunt. Semin Liver Dis 1999;19:457–73.

[35] Vangeli M, Patch D, Burroughs AK. Salvage TIPS for uncontrolled variceal bleeding. J Hepatol 2003;37:703–4.

[36] Jalan R, John TG, Redhead DN, et al. A comparative study of emergency transjugular intrahepatic portosystemic stent-shunt and esophageal transection in the management of uncontrolled variceal hemorrhage. Am J Gastroenterol 1995;90:1932–7.

[37] Smith JL, Graham DY. Variceal hemorrhage: a critical evaluation of survival analysis. Gastroenterology 1982;82:968–73.

[38] de Franchis R, Primignani M. Why do varices bleed? Gastroenterol Clin North Am 1992;21:85–101.

[39] Feu F, Garcia-Pagan JC, Bosch J, et al. Relation between portal pressure response to pharmacotherapy and risk of recurrent variceal haemorrhage in patients with cirrhosis. Lancet 1995;346:1056–9.

[40] Groszmann RJ, Bosch J, Grace ND, et al. Hemodynamic events in a prospective randomized trial of propanolol versus placebo in the prevention of a first variceal hemorrhage. Gastroenterology 1990;99:1401–7.

[41] Bernard B, Lebrec D, Mathurin P, et al. Beta-adrenergic antagonists in the prevention of gastrointestinal rebleeding in patients with cirrhosis: a meta-analysis. Hepatology 1997;25:63–70.

[42] Gournay J, Masliah C, Martin T, et al. Isosorbide mononitrate and propanolol compared with propanolol alone for the prevention of variceal rebleeding. Hepatology 2000;31:1239–45.

[43] Villanueva C, Balanzo J, Novella MT, et al. Nadolol plus isosorbide mononitratee compared with sclerotherapy for the prevention of variceal rebleeding. N Engl J Med 1996;334:1624–9.

[44] Villanueva C, Minana J, Ortiz J, et al. Endoscopic ligation compared with combined treatment with nadolol and isosorbide mononitrate to prevent recurrent variceal bleeding. N Engl J Med 2001;345:647–55.

[45] Lo GH, Chen WC, Chen MH, et al. Banding ligation versus nadolol and isosorbide mono-nitrate for the prevention of esophageal variceal rebleeding. Gastroenterology 2002;123: 728–34.

[46] Patch D, Sabin CA, Goulis J, et al. A randomized, controlled trial medical therapy versus endoscopic ligation for the prevention of variceal rebleeding in patients with cirrhosis. Gas-troenterology 2002;123:1013–9.

[47] Bernard B, Lebrec D, Mathurin P, et al. Propanolol and sclerotherapy in the prevention of gastrointestinal rebleeding in patients with cirrhosis. J Hepatol 1997;26:312–24.

[48] Laine L, Cook D. Endoscopic ligation compared with sclerotherapy for treatment of esoph-ageal variceal bleeding: a meta-analysis. Ann Intern Med 1995;123:280–7.

[49] Lo GH, Lai KH, Cheng JS, et al. Endoscopic variceal ligation plus nadolol and sucralfate compared with ligation alone for the prevention variceal rebleeding: a prospective random-ized trial. Hepatology 2000;32:461–5.

[50] de la Pena J, Brullet E, Sanchez-Hernandez E, et al. Variceal ligation plus nadolol compared with ligation for prophylaxis of variceal rebleeding: A multicenter trial. Hepatology 2005;41:572–8.

[51] Shaheen NJ, Stuart E, Schmitz S, et al. Pantoprazole reduces the size of postbanding ulcers after variceal band ligation: a randomized control trial. Hepatology 2005;41: 588–94.

[52] Spina GP, Henderson JM, Rikkers LF, et al. Distal spleno-renal shunt versus endoscopic scle-rotherapy in the prevention of variceal rebleeding. A meta-analysis of 4 randomized clinical trials. J Hepatol 1992;16(3):338–45.

[53] Papatheodoridis GV, Goulis J, Leandro G, et al. Transjugular intrahepatic portosystemic shunt compared with endoscopic treatment for prevention of variceal rebleeding: a meta-analysis. Hepatology 1999;30:612–22.

[54] Rosemurgy AS, Serafini FM, Zwebel BR, et al. Transjugular intrahepatic portosystemic shunt vs. small-diameter prosthetic H-graft portocaval shunt: Extended follow-up of an expanded randomized prospective trial. J Gastrointest Surg 2000;4:589–97.

[55] Thuluvath PJ, Yoo HY. Portal hypertensive gastropathy. Am J Gastroenterol 2002;97: 2973–8.

[56] McComrack TT, Sims J, Eyre-Brook I, et al. Gastric lesions in portal hypertension: inflamma-tory gastritis or congestive gastropathy? Gut 1985;26:1226–32.

[57] Primignani M, Carpinelli L, Preatoni P, et al. Natural history of portal hypertensive gastropa-thy in patients with liver cirrhosis. The New Italian Endoscopic Club for the study and treat-ment of esophageal varices (NIEC). Gastroenterology 2000;119:181–7.

[58] Merli M, Nicolini G, Angeloni S, et al. The natural history of portal hypertensive gastropathy in patients with liver cirrhosis and mild portal hypertension. Am J Gastroenterol 2004;99: 1959–65.

[59] Stewart CA, Sanyal AJ. Grading portal gastropathy: validation of a gastropathy scoring sys-tem. Am J Gastroenterol 2003;98:1758–65.

[60] Lebrec D, Ponyard T, Hillon P, et al. Propranolol for prevention of recurrent gastrointestinal bleeding in patients with cirrhosis. A controlled study. N Engl J Med 1981;305:1371–4.

[61] Hosking SW, Kennedy HJ, Seddon I, et al. The role of propranolol in congestive gastropathy of portal hypertension. Hepatology 1987;7:437–41.

[62] Perez-Ayuso RM, Pique JM, Bosch J, et al. Propranolol in prevention of recurrent bleeding from severe portal hypertension. Lancet 1991;337:1431–4.

[63] Kamath PS, Lacerda M, Ahlquist DA, et al. Gastric mucosal responses to intrahepatic porta-systemic shunting in patients with cirrhosis. Gastroenterology 2000;118:905–11.

[64] Spahr L, Villeneuve JP, Dufresne MP, et al. Gastric antral vascular ectasia in cirrhotic patients: absence of relation with portal hypertension. Gut 1999;44:739–42.

[65] Chalasani N, Kahi C, Francois F, et al. Outcomes following acute variceal bleeding: a mul-ticenter, cohort study. Am J Gastroenterol 2003;98:653–9.

[66] D'Amico G, De Franchis R. A cooperative study group. Upper digestive bleeding in cirrhosis. Post-therapeutic outcome and prognostic indicators. Hepatology 2003;38:599–612.

[67] Carbonell N, Pauwels A, Serfaty L, et al. Improved survival after variceal bleeding in patients with cirrhosis over the past two decades. Hepatology 2004;40:652–9.

[68] Sarin SK, Lahoti D, Saxena S, et al. Prevalence, classification and natural history of gastric varices: a long-term follow-up study in 568 portal hypertension patients. Hepatology 1992;16:1343.

[69] Greenwald BD, Caldwell SH, Hespenheide EE, et al. N-2-butyl-cyanoacrylate for bleeding gastric varices: a united states pilot study and cost analysis. Am J Gastroenterol 2003;98:1982–8.

[70] Kind R, Guglielmi A, Rodella L, et al. Bucrylate treatment of bleeding gastric varices: 12 years experience. Endoscopy 2000;32:512–9.

[71] Lo GH, Lai KH, Cheng JS, et al. A prospective randomized trial of butyl cyanoacrylate injection versus band ligation in the management of bleeding gastric varices. Hepatology 2001;33:1060–4.

[72] Huang YH, Yeh HZ, Chen GH, et al. Endoscopic treatment of bleeding gastric varices by N-2-cyanoacrylate (histoacryl) injection: long-term efficacy and safety. Gastrointest Endosc 2000;52:160–7.

[73] Barange K, Peron JM, Imani K, et al. Transjugular intrahepatic portasystemic shunt in the treatment of refractory bleeding from ruptured gastric varices. Hepatology 1999;30:1139–43.

[74] Tripathi D, Therapondos G, Jackson E, et al. The role of the transjugular intrahepatic portasystemic stent shunt (TIPSS) in the management of bleeding gastric varices: clinical and haemodynamic correlations. Gut 2002;51:270–4.

[75] Kanagawa H, Mima S, Kouyama H, et al. Treatment of gastric fundal varices by balloon-occluded retrograde transvenous obliteration. J Gastroenterol Hepatol 1996;11:51–8.

[76] Chikamori F, Kuniyoshi N, Shibuya S, et al. Eight years experience with transjugular retrograde obliteration for gastric varices with gastro–renal shunts. Surgery 2001;129:414–20.

[77] Tomikawa M, Hashizume M, Saku M, et al. Effectiveness of gastric devascularization and splenectomy for patients with gastric varices. J Am Coll Surg 2000;191:498–503.

[78] Orloff MJ, Orloff MS, Girard B, et al. Bleeding esophagogastric varices from extrahepatic portal hypertension: 40 years' experience with portal-systemic shunt. J Am Coll Surg 2002;194:717–28.

[79] Shiba M, Higuchi K, Nagamura K, et al. Efficacy and safety of balloon-occluded endoscopic injection therapy as a prophylactic treatment for high-risk gastric fundal varices: a prospective, randomized, comparative trial. Gastrointest Endosc 2002;56:522–8.

[80] Rengstorff DS, Binmoeller KF. A pilot study of 2-octyl cyanoacrylate injection for treatment of gastric fundal varices in humans. Gastrointest Endosc 2004;59:553–8.

[81] Grace ND. Diagnosis and treatment of gastrointestinal bleeding secondary to portal hypertension. Am J Gastroenterol 1997;92:1081–91.

[82] Grace ND, Groszmann RJ, Garcia-Tsao G, et al. Portal hypertension and variceal bleeding: an AASLD single topic symposium. Hepatology 1998;28:868–80.

[83] de Franchis R. Evolving consensus in portal hypertension. Report of the Baveno IV consensus workshop on methodology of diagnosis and therapy in portal hypertension. J Hepatol 2005;43:167–76.

[84] D'Amico G, Morabito A. Noninvasive markers of esophageal varices: another round, not the last. Hepatology 2004;39:30–4.

[85] Boyer TD, Henderson MJ. Portal hypertension and bleeding esophageal varices. In: Boyer AD, editor. Hepatology: a text book of hepatology. 4th edition. Philadelphia: Elsevier Science; 2003. p. 581–629.

[86] Boyer TD. Changing clinical practice with measurements of portal pressure. Hepatology 2004;39:283–5.

[87] Groszmann R, Wongcharatawee S. The hepatic venous pressure gradient: anything worth doing should be done right. Hepatology 2004;39:280–2.

[88] Abraczinskas DR, Ookubo R, Grace ND, et al. Propranolol for the prevention of first esophageal variceal hemorrhage: a lifetime commitment? Hepatology 2001;34:1092–102.

[89] Imperiale TF, Chalasani NA. Meta-analysis of endoscopic variceal ligation in primary prophylaxis of esophageal variceal bleeding in patients with cirrhosis. Hepatology 2001;33: 821–5.

[90] Khuroo MS, Khuroo NS, Farahat KLC, et al. Meta-analysis: endoscopic variceal ligation for primary prophylaxis of oesophageal variceal bleeding. Aliment Pharmacol Ther 2005;21: 347–61.

[91] Merkel C, Marin R, Angeli P, et al. A placebo-controlled clinical trial of nadolol in the prophylaxis of growth of small esophageal varices in cirrhosis. Gastroenterology 2004;127: 476–84.

[92] Groszmann RJ, Garcia-Tsao G, Makuch R, et al. Multi-center randomized placebo-controlled trial of non-selective beta-blockers in the prevention of the complications of portal hypertension: final results and identification of a predictive factor. Hepatology 2003;38:206A.

[93] Arguedas MR, Heudebert GR, Eloubedi MA, et al. Cost-effectiveness of screening, surveillance and primary prophylaxis strategies for esophageal varices. Am J Gastroenterol 2002;97:2441–52.

[94] Saab SM, DeRosa V, Nieto J, et al. Costs and clinical outcomes for primary prophylaxis of varices; bleeding in patients with hepatic cirrhosis: a decision analytic model. Am J Gastroenterol 2003;98:763–70.

[95] Spiegel BMR, Targowik L, Dulai GS, et al. Endoscopic screening for esophageal varices: is it ever cost effective? Hepatology 2003;37:366–77.

[96] Cales P, Oberti F, Payen JL, et al. Lack of effect of propranolol in the prevention of large oesophageal varices in patients with cirrhosis: a randomized trial. French-Speaking Club for the Study of Portal Hypertension. Eur J Gastroenterol Hepatol 1999;11:741–5.

Gastroenterol Clin N Am 34 (2005) 643–664

GASTROENTEROLOGY CLINICS
OF NORTH AMERICA

Lower GI Bleeding: Epidemiology and Diagnosis

Lisa L. Strate, MD, MPH[a,b,*]

[a]Harvard Medical School, Boston, MA 02115, USA
[b]Division of Gastroenterology, Brigham and Women's Hospital, 75 Francis Street, Boston, MA 02115, USA

Lower gastrointestinal bleeding (LGIB) is anatomically defined as bleeding beyond the ligament of Treitz. The term "lower gastrointestinal bleeding" is therefore a misnomer, and a more appropriate term would be lower intestinal bleeding. Clinically, LGIB represents a diverse range of bleeding sources and severities, ranging from scant hemorrhoidal bleeding to massive blood loss from vascular small bowel tumors. Various terms are used to describe blood emanating from the lower intestinal tract, including hematochezia, rectal bleeding, and bright red blood per rectum. These terms do not indicate the acuity or severity of bleeding, do not always localize the bleeding source, and are not exclusive to bleeding from beyond the ligament of Treitz. The wide clinical spectrum of LGIB and the number of available management strategies present a challenge for clinicians and investigators both. This review focuses on the epidemiology and diagnosis of acute LGIB with an emphasis on bleeding from colonic sources.

EPIDEMIOLOGY
Incidence

Acute LGIB is one of the most common gastrointestinal indications for hospital admission. The annual incidence of hospitalization for LGIB was estimated to be 20 to 30 per 100,000 persons in a large, southern California health maintenance organization [1]. This rate increased dramatically with advancing age [1]. Consequently, the impact of this disorder promises to increase as the population ages. In comparison, in the same population, the annual incidence of hospitalization for acute upper gastrointestinal bleeding (UGIB) was 100 per 100,000 persons per year [2]. Other studies also indicate that LGIB is approximately one-fifth as common as UGIB [3–5].

The author is supported by a grant (K08 HS014062-01) from the Agency for Healthcare Research and Quality, Rockville, MD.

*Division of Gastroenterology, Brigham and Women's Hospital, 75 Francis Street, Boston, MA 02115, USA. E-mail address: lstrate@partners.org

Demographics

Lower gastrointestinal bleeding predominantly afflicts an older population with a mean age of more than 65 years in most studies [5–11]. The annual incidence rate of hospitalization increases from 1 per 100,000 patients in the third decade of life to over 200 per 100,000 in patients in the ninth decade [1]. The older age distribution reflects the most common causes of LGIB (eg, diverticulosis, ischemic colitis) that tend to occur with aging. Concurrent with the older age distribution is a significant burden of comorbid illness. Studies reveal that at least 70% of patients with LGIB have at least one coexistent condition (see Refs. [6,10,12,13]).

In the population-based study of LGIB by Longstreth, men were affected significantly more frequently than women [1]. Little information exists regarding racial differences in LGIB. Diverticular disease, the most common cause of LGIB in the United States, is primarily a disease of Western cultures. However, this geographic variation is highly influenced by diet and lifestyle factors [14].

Outcomes

Most patients with LGIB have favorable outcomes despite advanced age and comorbid conditions [15,16]. Major outcomes and their frequency are listed in Table 1. Mortality rates range from 0% to 25% (see Refs. [1,17–19]). Mortality rates greater than 5% are generally found in older studies of severely bleeding patients in which a high percentage underwent emergency surgery [18–20]. As in UGIB, patients who begin bleeding while hospitalized for a separate disease process (inpatient bleeding) have a significantly higher risk of death than those who are admitted with LGIB (23% versus 2.4%) [1]. Most deaths are not the direct result of uncontrolled bleeding but rather exacerbation of an

Table 1
Outcomes of acute lower gastrointestinal bleeding

First author/Year	n	Acute rebleeding[a] (%)	Delayed rebleeding (%)	Surgery (%)	Mortality (%)	PRBC[b] (mean units)	Length of stay (mean days)
Schmulewitz 2003 [10]	565	11	12	5	3	3.1	6.7
Das 2003 [8]	332	19	—	—	5	2.2	4.4
Strate 2003 [11,12]	252	7	—	4	2	2	4.3
Longstreth 1997 [1]	219	—	16	16	4	—	—
McGuire[c] 1994 [23]	118	24	38	24	3	3.2	—
Richter 1995 [24]	107	25	—	8	1	4	11
Angtuaco 2001 [22]	90	13	—	6	2	—	4
Chaudhry 1998 [7]	85	32	12	11	4	1.8	—

[a] Persistent hemorrhage or recurrent bleeding during the initial hospitalization. Definitions vary across studies.
[b] Packed red blood cells.
[c] Diverticular bleeding only.

underlying disorder or development of a nosocomial complication (see Refs. [1,11,21]). However, all-cause mortality during long-term follow-up is substantial. In a population-based study with 3 years of follow-up, death occurred in 19% of patients. Increasing age, duration of hospital stay, and number of comorbid conditions were independent predictors of all-cause mortality [1].

Most patients with LGIB will stop bleeding spontaneously. Continued or recurrent bleeding during an acute episode occurs in 10% to 40% of patients (see Refs. [1,7,8,10,11,22–24]). Between 5% and 50% of patients with persistent bleeding require surgical hemostasis (see Refs. [7,8,11,17,22,25]). Advances in endoscopic and radiologic hemostasis techniques appear to be decreasing rates of surgical intervention and rebleeding [13,26]. Long-term recurrence is a particular problem for patients with bleeding from diverticulosis or angiodysplasia [1,16]. These disorders will be discussed in subsequent sections.

The economic burden of LGIB on the whole has not been formally assessed but is presumably significant given the prevalence of this disorder and the older, often debilitated, patient population. Using the National Inpatient Sample, the largest, nationwide inpatient database, Thomas and colleagues estimated that diverticular hemorrhage alone cost $1.3 billion in 2001 [27]. In a study of acute LGIB in Ontario, Canada, the average cost for a patient with LGIB was $4,832 Canadian dollars (approximately $3,000 US) with an average length of stay of 7.5 days [28].

Predicting Outcome

Extensive literature exists regarding risk stratification in UGIB. Until recently, little was known about predictors of outcome in LGIB. The BLEED classification system (ongoing bleeding, systolic blood pressure less than 100 mmHg, prothrombin time greater than 1.2 times control, altered mental status, and unstable comorbid disease) was designed to stratify patients with either upper or lower gastrointestinal hemorrhage according to their risk of adverse in-hospital events [3,29]. Das and colleagues developed and validated artificial neural networks (ANNs) for the prediction of recurrent bleeding, need for intervention and death in the context of LGIB [8]. These ANN-based models were highly accurate, particularly when compared with the BLEED classification, and outperformed standard regression models when tested in an external cohort. Strate and colleagues identified seven independent predictors of severity in acute LGIB (hypotension, tachycardia, syncope, nontender abdominal exam, bleeding within 4 hours of presentation, aspirin use, and more than two comorbid diseases) [40]. Based on these factors, patients could be stratified into three risk groups: Patients with more than three risk factors had an 84% risk of severe bleeding, one to three risk factors a 43% risk, and no risk factors a 9% risk. These findings were prospectively validated in a mixed cohort of patients from an academic and a community hospital [30]. Velayos and colleagues prospectively studied patients admitted with LGIB and identified three predictors of severity and adverse outcome (initial hematocrit less than 35%, abnormal vital signs, and gross blood on rectal exam) [5]. Ideally, these predictive tools will help guide the initial triage of patients with LGIB and a more standardized and cost-effective approach to this disorder.

DIAGNOSIS

Diagnostic Criteria

Multiple factors make the identification of a precise bleeding source in LGIB challenging. These include the diversity of potential sources, the length of bowel involved, the need for colon cleansing, and the intermittent nature of bleeding. In up to 40% of patients with LGIB, more than one potential bleeding source will be noted [31], and stigmata of recent bleeding in LGIB are infrequently identified (see Refs. [12,13,17]). As a result, no definitive source will be found in a large percentage of patients (see Refs. [6,10,32]). Various authors have attempted to define criteria for diagnosis in LGIB (see Refs. [1,16,33]), but these criteria have not been used consistently. Standardization of reporting on LGIB using such criteria would improve the quality of research and clinical care, as well as our understanding of the epidemiology of this disorder.

Clinical History

A thorough history and physical exam should be part of the initial evaluation of all patients presenting with gastrointestinal bleeding and can be done simultaneous with resuscitation efforts. The duration, frequency, and color of blood passed per rectum may help discern the severity and location of bleeding. Characteristically, melena or black, tarry stool, indicates bleeding from an upper gastrointestinal or small bowel source, whereas bright red blood per rectum signifies bleeding from the left colon or rectum. However, patient and physician reports of stool color are often inaccurate and inconsistent [34]. In addition, even with objectively defined bright red bleeding, significant proximal lesions can be found on colonoscopy [35].

The past medical history may also help to elucidate a specific bleeding source. Key points include antecedent constipation or diarrhea (hemorrhoids, colitis), the presence of diverticulosis (diverticular bleeding), receipt of radiation therapy (radiation enteritis), recent polypectomy (postpolypectomy bleeding), and vascular disease/hypotension (ischemic colitis). A family history of colon cancer increases the likelihood of a colorectal neoplasm and generally calls for a complete colonic examination in patients with hematochezia. Nonetheless, even after a detailed history, physicians cannot reliably predict which patients with hematochezia will have significant pathology [36], and a history of bleeding from one source does not eliminate the possibility of bleeding from a different source.

Physical Examination

A thorough physical examination is important to assess blood volume loss, a possible bleeding source, and comorbid conditions (which may affect suitability for interventions such as urgent colonoscopy). Orthostatic vital signs are an important complement to standard monitoring in a patient with apparently severe bleeding but without overt hemodynamic instability. The presence of abdominal tenderness on examination may indicate an inflammatory disorder, such as ischemic colitis or inflammatory bowel disease, in contrast with a vascular source, such as diverticula or angiodysplasia [11]. The rectal exam serves to identify anorectal lesions and confirm stool color. However, positive findings on rectal examination do not preclude a concomitant abnormal finding on colonoscopy [37]. Despite presenting features and findings on physical examination, most patients with LGIB warrant a full examination of the colon.

Exclusion of an Upper Gastrointestinal Source

Several tools in addition to stool color are used to discriminate upper from lower gastrointestinal bleeding. This is an important step because 2% to 15% of patients with presumed LGIB will have UGIB [9]. Nasogastric lavage is a quick and safe procedure, but to avoid unnecessary patient discomfort, it should be reserved for patients with evidence of brisk bleeding in whom an upper endoscopy is not anticipated. Nasogastric lavage containing gross blood, 25% blood-tinged fluid, or strongly guaiac positive dark fluid was found to have 80% sensitivity for bleeding above the ligament of Treitz, and positive and negative predictive values of 93% and 99%, respectively [38]. Some authors believe that the presence of bile increases the sensitivity of nasogastric lavage [9], although the correlation between a bilious appearing aspirate and the true presence of bile acids has been questioned [39]. A nasogastric tube may also aid in the administration of a rapid bowel preparation [13] and should, ideally, be left in place until management decisions have been made. The blood urea nitrogen to creatinine ratio is a noninvasive test also used to help distinguish upper versus colonic sources of bleeding [40–42]. In one study, a ratio of 33 or higher had a sensitivity of 96% for UGIB, although overlap was observed with LGIB, especially in patients with UGIB without hematemesis [40]. Esophagoduodenoscopy remains the gold standard for excluding an UGI source in patients presenting with severe bleeding, especially those with hemodynamic instability.

DIAGNOSTIC PROCEDURES

Colonoscopy

Advances in endoscopic technology have brought colonoscopy to the forefront of the management of LGIB. Recent studies have shown that colonoscopy, particularly when performed early (within 12 to 24 hours of admission), is safe and effective (see Refs. [7,9,12,13,31]). Colonoscopy is undoubtedly the best test for confirming the source of LGIB and for excluding ominous diagnoses, such as malignancy. The diagnostic yield of colonoscopy ranges from 45% to 95% (Table 2) [6,13]. Discrepancies in diagnostic rates are at least in part the result of the criteria (or lack of) used to confirm a bleeding source (ie, probable versus definitive). In general, comparisons across studies are difficult because of variability in study design, patient selection, timing of exams, bowel preparation, and endoscopic experience.

Various therapeutic interventions (which are discussed in the subsequent chapter) are possible with colonoscopy; therefore, it is an efficient and

Table 2
Colonoscopy for the diagnosis of lower gastrointestinal bleeding

First author/Year	n	Diagnosis (%)	Definite diagnosis (%)	Complete exam (%)	Complications (%)
Less than 12 hours from admission:					
Jensen 2000 [13]	121	96	88	—	1[a]
Jensen 1988 [9]	80	74	74	100	5
Less than 24 hours from admission:					
Ohyama[b] 2000 [89]	345	89	—	56	0
Chaudhry[b] 1998 [7]	85	97	—	68	1
Angtuaco 2001 [22]	39	75	8	—	—
Caos 1986 [31]	35	77	63	—	0
More than 24 hours from admission or no time specified:					
Schmulewitz 2003 [10]	415	89	—	—	0.2
Tada[b] 1991 [46]	206	89	—	59	—
Wang 1991 [112]	205	94	73	66	0
Al Qahtani 2002 [6]	152	45	—	87	—
Strate 2003 [12]	144	89	43	—	1
Richter 1995 [24]	78	90	60	73	0
Colacchio 1982 [47]	58	48	—	—	2
Vellacott 1986 [49]	21	67	—	33	0

[a] One pneumonia not noted to be related to endoscopy.
[b] No colon preparation. In the Ohyama study, no preparation for patients studied from 1976 to 1990; from 1990 to 1995, polyethylene glycol solution used.

presumably cost-effective approach to most patients with LGIB. Early performance of colonoscopy has been shown to reduce length of hospital stay independent of other factors, such as severity of bleeding and comorbid illness (see Refs. [10,12,24,43]) and therefore should decrease treatment costs [44,45]. Reduction in length of stay appears to be related to establishing low-risk diagnoses rather than performance of therapeutic interventions [12]. In comparison, most patients undergoing radiographic evaluation for LGIB regardless of findings and interventions will subsequently require a colonoscopy to establish the cause of bleeding.

The optimal timing of colonoscopic intervention for LGIB remains uncertain. Early reports of emergency colonoscopy designated 24 hours from admission as the time threshold [7,46], whereas more recent literature defines urgent colonoscopy as within 12 hours [9,13]. Evidence suggests, although not overwhelmingly, that earlier performance leads to more diagnostic and therapeutic opportunities [13,47] and reduces length of stay (see Refs. [10,12,24,43]). However, urgent colonoscopy is difficult to orchestrate, and logistical factors, such as time of admission, appear to play a significant role in determining whether a patient will undergo endoscopic or radiographic intervention [48]. A good bowel preparation is important for the adequacy and sensitivity of urgent colonoscopy but is challenging for nursing staff and patients. Early reports of unprepped colonoscopy for LGIB report completion rates as low as 35%

[46,49] compared with 100% in a study using aggressive purges [13]. In the later study, preparation entailed 5 to 6 liters of sulfate purge, and nasogastric tubes in 33% of participants [13]. However, adequate and safe cleansing has been reported using less aggressive measures [31]. Around-the-clock endoscopy facilities and support staff also help to facilitate timely exams, but are not available in all hospitals.

Traditionally, colonoscopic evaluation for LGIB was delayed because of the need for adequate bowel preparation and the fear of increased procedural risks. Indeed urgent colonoscopy in an unprepped colon can be challenging if not dangerous. However, complication rates for colonoscopy in LGIB are low, and bowel preparation itself appears to be safe [31]. Zuckerman and Prakash, in a review of 13 studies, found an overall complication rate of 1.3% [50]. The most commonly reported complications are fluid overload [7,9], bowel perforation (see Refs. [7,10,47,51]), and sepsis [49].

Radionuclide Scintigraphy

Localization of the bleeding source is an important challenge in the management of LGIB. Radionuclide scintigraphy is a method that has been used for this purpose since the 1970s. Two methods exist—one using technetium-99m (Tc-99m) sulfur colloid and the other Tc-99m-labeled red blood cells (tagged red blood cell scan). Sulfur colloid is simple to prepare and is rapidly cleared from the circulation. However, uptake in the spleen, liver, and bone marrow compromise localization of UGIB sources. Radiolabeled red blood cells have a longer half-life, making it possible to perform repeat scans for recurrent bleeding following a single injection. In addition, red cell scans may localize bleeding anywhere outside the splenic area. Despite these theoretical advantages, a comparison of these two techniques found no difference in bleeding detection rates [52].

Among the advantages of radionuclide scanning are its sensitivity for bleeding as low as 0.05 to 0.1 ml/min [53] and its noninvasive nature. In addition, no bowel preparation is required, venous and arterial bleeding can both be detected, and repeat scans can be easily performed in the event of recurrent bleeding. However, radionuclide scanning has variable accuracy, cannot confirm the source of bleeding, and may delay other diagnostic and therapeutic procedures. Therefore, the role of radionuclide scintigraphy in the evaluation of patients with LGIB remains controversial.

Radionuclide scintigraphy is advocated for two primary purposes—as a guide for surgical resection and as a screening test prior to angiography. However, there is wide variability in the reported accuracy and usefulness of radionuclide scintigraphy for these purposes (Table 3) (see Refs. [19–21,54–64]). Radionuclide scintigraphy in some series accurately localized bleeding in more than 90% of patients undergoing emergency surgery [65]. However, other authors describe poor accuracy and a high rate of false positive exams [56,62]. In one study, 42% of patients underwent an incorrect surgical procedure based on scintigraphy results [56]. In addition, several studies have found that regardless of accuracy, scintigraphy did not affect surgical management (see Refs.

Table 3
Radionuclide scintigraphy for the diagnosis of lower gastrointestinal bleeding

First author/Year	Total scans	Positive scans (%)	Bleeding site confirmed (%)	Correct localization[a] (%)	Angiography in patients with positive scans (%)	Positive angiograms (%)
Levy 2003 [20]	287	70	95	47	20	0
Suzman 1996 [21]	224	51	32	78[b]	14	44
Hunter 1990 [56]	203	26	42	41	—	—
Ng 1997 [59]	160	54	—	—	55	43
Gutierrez 1998 [113]	105	40	60	88	—	—
Winn 1983 [63]	82	16	92	100	62	38
Rantis 1995 [61]	80	48	58	73	50	—
Orecchia 1985 [60]	76	34	62	94	—	—
Kester 1984 [57]	62	60	24	67	24	22
Voeller 1991 [62]	59	32	84	69	—	—
Markisz 1982 [58]	50	34	65	91	65	36
Alavi 1980[c] [54]	43	54	91	48	100	43
Nicholson 1989 [114]	43	72	97	97	—	—
Winzelberg 1981 [65]	32	91	90	96	90	39
Leitman 1989 [19]	28	43	—	86	100	50

[a] Of those patients who had confirmation of the bleeding site.
[b] Localization was 87% if segmental localization versus precise localization was used.
[c] Tc-99m sulfur colloid. Other studies in table used Tc-99m-labeled red blood cells.

[20,62,66]). Accuracy appears to be best when the scan becomes positive within a short period of time (see Refs. [57,60,65]).

A similar debate exists with regard to the usefulness of radionuclide scintigraphy as a screening test for angiography. In theory, this noninvasive and more sensitive test would be used to select patients for angiography and to guide selective contrast injections. Gunderman and colleagues found that the yield of angiography increased from 22% to 53% after implementation of screening radionuclide scintigraphy [67]. In addition, several studies demonstrate that angiography following a negative radionuclide scan is of low yield [54,58]. However, in other series screening, radionuclide scintigraphy did not increase the rate of positive angiograms [68,69] and potentially delayed other therapeutic interventions [18].

These discrepancies regarding radionuclide scintigraphy may be attributed to several factors. First, selection criteria for studies vary with regard to severity and location of bleeding. Radionuclide scintigraphy is presumably most sensitive to severe bleeding and more accurate for lower gastrointestinal sources (excluding the rectum) (see Refs. [21,54,62,68,70]). Second, criteria for bleeding localization and site confirmation differ across studies. Some studies require precise localization and surgical confirmation, whereas others have much less rigorous criteria. In addition, imaging techniques in the literature are not standardized. Real-time, continuous dynamic imaging appears to be superior to delayed static imaging [70]. Last, the time to scan positivity [59,71], and the delay before angiography [18], may influence results but are infrequently noted. Prospective, randomized studies of radionuclide scanning in the management of LGIB would help resolve questions regarding its usefulness.

Angiography

Angiography is another radiographic modality used in the management of LGIB. Angiography is less sensitive than radionuclide scanning with the ability to detect bleeding of more than 0.5 ml/min [72]. In addition to its diagnostic role, angiography offers therapeutic possibilities via pharmacologic vasoconstriction or selective microembolization, and therefore may reduce the need for surgical resection. Disadvantages of angiography for LGIB include the potential for serious complications, the need for active bleeding at the time of the exam, and the need for confirmation of the bleeding source.

Bleeding detection rates with angiography range from 20% to 70% (Table 4) (see Refs. [19,47,54,59,69,73–75]). Severity of bleeding at the time of angiography is ostensibly related to the sensitivity of this exam [18,66,69]. Other factors that may affect the sensitivity of angiography include intermittent bleeding, procedural delays, atherosclerotic anatomy, and venous or small vessel bleeding [69,73]. Variability in patient selection and radiographic techniques may account for disparate results across studies. In addition, technologic advances in coaxial catheter and embolization technology have improved the ability to localize and treat LGIB over time.

Angiography has traditionally been used to guide surgical resection [73,74]. Segmental resection is reported in 50% to 95% of patients with positive angiograms (see Table 4) [18,74,75]. However, this represents only 10% to 60% of all patients undergoing angiography. As many as 20% to 50% of patients with negative angiograms will also require surgery [74,75]. Recurrent bleeding following angiographic-guided segmental resection appears to be low. In a collective series of 167 patients, rebleeding occurred in 6% [73]. Vasopressin

Table 4
Angiography for the diagnosis of lower gastrointestinal bleeding

First author/Year	Total no.	Positive (%)	Guided segmental surgical resection (%)	Complications (%)
Pennoyer 1997 [69]	131	34	—	3
Colacchio 1982 [47]	98	41	—	4
Cohn 1998 [75]	75	35	12	11
Leitman 1989 [19]	68	40	—	10
Caserella 1974 [74]	60	67	50	—
Browder 1996 [73]	50	72	34	—
Ng 1997 [59]	47	43	—	6
Alavi 1981 [54]	43	23	—	—

infusion may also be used to stabilize patients, allowing for more elective and safer surgery [73]. However, advances in supraselective embolization techniques appear to be replacing vasopressin infusion and decreasing the need for surgical intervention [26].

Complications occur in 0% to 10% of patients undergoing angiography, although adverse events are inconsistently reported in the literature. The most common complications appear to be hematoma or bleeding at the catheter site (see Refs. [47,69,75]). Other potential adverse events include arterial dissection, catheter site infection, loss of pedal pulses, and contrast reaction (see Refs. [47,69,75]). Myocardial and intestinal ischemia, renal failure, and cardiac arrhythmias have been reported with the use of vasopressin infusion (see Refs. [19,43,76]). Localized bowel ischemia and infarction are concerns with therapeutic embolization [19,76]. Technologic advances in coaxial catheter techniques, embolization materials, and nonionic contrast agents promise to reduce complication rates in diagnostic and therapeutic angiography.

Infusion of vasodilators, anticoagulants, and thrombolytics can be used to provoke bleeding prior to angiography in patients with intractable bleeding of unknown origin. Using these techniques, bleeding is detected in 20% to 80% of patients [77–79]. Complications, including hematoma and continued bleeding, occur in 0% to 20% of patients [78]. Data regarding these techniques is limited to small series of patients, and severe complications, including intracranial hemorrhage and uncontrolled bleeding, are possible. Optimal results may depend on technical expertise, type and dosage of provocative agents, and timing of intervention in relation to onset of bleeding [77]. Experienced operators and carefully selected patients are necessary to achieve good results and limit complications [77]. Capsule endoscopy is currently a safer and promising diagnostic test for bleeding of unknown origin, and may obviate the need for provocative angiography in some of these difficult patients.

Studies directly comparing outcomes of radiographic versus colonoscopic interventions for LGIB are limited. Jensen and colleagues performed urgent colonoscopy (less than 12 hours from admission) and angiography on 22 patients with severe bleeding. The diagnostic yield of colonoscopy was 82% compared with 12% for angiography [43]. In a prospective trial of 100 patients randomized to colonoscopy within 8 hours or radionuclide scintigraphy followed by angiography, colonoscopy yielded significantly more diagnoses [80]. No differences were seen in therapeutic interventions, mortality, surgery, blood transfusions, or length of stay. However, there was a trend in favor of colonoscopy, and the study was not adequately powered for these outcomes. The advantages and disadvantages of frequently used interventions for LGIB are outlined in Table 5.

Other Diagnostic Modalities for LGIB

Flexible sigmoidoscopy can be performed expediently and may play a role in the initial evaluation of patients with LGIB [31]. The diagnostic yield of flexible sigmoidoscopy in LGIB ranges from 9% to 58% (see Refs. [6,12,24,35,47,49]).

Table 5
Advantages and disadvantages of common diagnostic procedures used in the evaluation of lower gastrointestinal bleeding

Procedure	Advantages	Disadvantages
Colonoscopy	• Therapeutic possibilities • Diagnostic for all sources of bleeding • Needed to confirm diagnosis in most patients regardless of initial testing • Efficient/cost-effective	• Bowel preparation required • Can be difficult to orchestrate without on-call endoscopy facilities or staff • Invasive
Angiography	• No bowel preparation needed • Therapeutic possibilities • May be superior for patients with severe bleeding	• Requires active bleeding at the time of the exam • Less sensitive to venous bleeding • Diagnosis must be confirmed with endoscopy/surgery • Serious complications are possible
Radionuclide scintigraphy	• Noninvasive • Sensitive to low rates of bleeding • No bowel preparation • Easily repeated if bleeding recurs	• Variable accuracy (false positives) • Not therapeutic • May delay therapeutic intervention • Diagnosis must be confirmed with endoscopy/surgery
Flexible sigmoidoscopy	• Diagnostic and therapeutic • Minimal bowel preparation • Easy to perform	• Visualizes only the left colon • Colonoscopy or other test usually necessary to rule out right-sided lesions

In studies with favorable results, patients with a high suspicion of a left colon source were preferentially triaged to this strategy [35]. Therapeutic interventions for stigmata of active bleeding are also possible. However, regardless of presentation, flexible sigmoidoscopy may miss serious proximal pathology [35]. Fine and colleagues studied 217 patients with acute or subacute bright red blood per rectum [35]. Eight were found to have proximal cancers, three of which were in young patients without a family history of colorectal cancer. Unless a definite and compatible bleeding source is identified with flexible sigmoidoscopy, workup should proceed with a full colonoscopy in most patients.

With the advent of improved endoscopic technology, barium enema is uncommonly used in the evaluation of LGIB. Barium enema cannot detect superficial lesions or confirm a definitive bleeding source and may miss important pathology [47,81]. In one study, 79 of 173 patients (46%) undergoing barium enema were found to have significant lesions at colonoscopy, including 20 malignancies [81]. Furthermore, barium contrast may complicate subsequent colonoscopy or angiography. Contrast-enhanced computed tomography (CT) and magnetic resonance (MR) angiography are newer radiographic techniques that show promise in the evaluation of lower gastrointestinal bleeding and also offer the diagnostic capabilities of cross-sectional imaging [82,83].

Small bowel evaluation is indicated when upper and lower endoscopies fail to identify a source of bleeding. Traditionally, push enteroscopy and small bowel contrast radiography were the procedures of choice. Capsule endoscopy is the newest technology for evaluation of the gastrointestinal tract and plays a clear role in patients with small intestinal or obscure gastrointestinal bleeding. The diagnostic yield in patients with overt bleeding and negative upper and lower endoscopies ranges from 40% to 90% [84,85]. Capsule endoscopy has proven superior to other modalities used for obscure gastrointestinal bleeding. The diagnostic yield of capsule endoscopy ranges from 55% to 70% versus 25% to 30% for push endoscopy [86,87]. Costamagna and colleagues found that a source of obscure bleeding was found in 31% of patients with capsule endoscopy, and only 5% with barium small bowel radiographs [88]. Colonic sources of bleeding are difficult to evaluate via capsule endoscopy because of retained stool, limited battery life, and poor field of vision due to the colon's large diameter. Technological advancements in capsule endoscopy are likely to improve diagnostic accuracy and may facilitate procedural interventions.

SOURCES OF BLEEDING

Lower gastrointestinal bleeding arises from a diverse range of sources. Table 6 displays the breakdown of sources from a number of large studies. The spectrum of sources appears to be changing over time [16,89]. In the early 20th century, neoplasia was reported as the predominant source of LGIB, and diverticular bleeding was presumably rare [16]. Angiodysplasia were increasingly recognized as a source of LGIB in the 1960s and 1970s [16]. Currently, diverticular bleeding is the leading source of LGIB. This evolving disease spectrum may reflect a true change in the epidemiology of LGIB as well as improvements in diagnostic techniques and criteria. Common sources of LGIB are briefly discussed in the following sections.

Diverticular Bleeding

Diverticular disease currently comprises 20% to 55% of all cases of LGIB (see Refs. [1,10,11,13,46,89]). Diverticulosis is rare in patients under 40 years of age, but is seen in up to 65% of patients over the age of 85 [90]. It is estimated that 3% to 15% of patients with diverticulosis will experience bleeding [25]. Patients with diverticular hemorrhage typically present with the sudden onset of hematochezia and signs and symptoms of significant blood loss. Most patients will stop bleeding spontaneously, but up to 25% will require emergent intervention [25]. Stigmata of recent hemorrhage are infrequently identified [17] but appear to predict recurrent bleeding and the need for surgery in a manner similar to stigmata in UGIB (Fig. 1) [13].

The etiology and pathophysiology of diverticular bleeding is incompletely understood but may be the result of repeated trauma to the vasa recta (nutrient

Table 6
Sources of lower gastrointestinal bleeding

Source	Schmulewitz [10] (1993–2000) (%)	Ohyama [89] (1976–1995) (%)	Strate [12] (1996–1999) (%)	Longstreth [1] (1990–1993) (%)	Tada [47] (1975–1991) (%)
Diverticulosis	35	5	30	42	8
Ischemia	6	18	10	9	17
Anorectal[a]	12	9	16	6	16
Neoplasia[b]	7	3	6	9	11
Angiodysplasia	3	1	3	3	0
Postpolypectomy	3	13	7	4	0
IBD[c]	3	2	4	3	—
Colitis, other[d]	3	24	8	6	29
Radiation colitis	2	—	3	1	—
Small bowel/ UGIB	5	5	—	3	13
Other	1	9	5	2	2
Unknown	23	11	9	12	6
Total	565	345	252	219	206

Probable and definitive sources.
[a]Anorectal sources include hemorrhoids, anal fissures, rectal/stercoral ulcers.
[b]Neoplasia includes polyps and cancers.
[c]Inflammatory bowel disease (ulcerative colitis and Crohn's disease).
[d]Infectious colitis, antibiotic associated colitis, colitis of unclear etiology.

arteries) that stretch over the diverticular dome. Nonsteroidal anti-inflammatory drugs have shown an association with diverticular complications in several prospective studies [91,92]. Advancing age and right-sided location may also play a role (see Refs. [1,74,93]). Long-term recurrence rates for diverticular bleeding increase from 9% at 1 year to 48% at 10 years [1,93]. After the second episode of bleeding, there is a 50% chance of recurrence [93]. Severity of the index bleed does not appear to predict recurrence [93]. Empiric preventative measures include a high-fiber diet and avoidance of nonsteroidal anti-inflammatories.

Ischemic Colitis

Colonic ischemia is the most common form of intestinal ischemia and in most cases is transient and reversible. This is in contrast to acute mesenteric ischemia, which is a medical emergency. The colon is predisposed to ischemic insult because of its poor collateral circulation, low blood flow, and high bacterial content. The watershed areas of the splenic flexure, rectosigmoid junction, and right colon are commonly involved because of their particularly tenuous blood supply.

Colonic ischemia should be considered in patients presenting with the sudden onset of abdominal pain and bloody diarrhea. Any event or condition that compromises colonic blood flow can lead to ischemia, although most patients have no identifiable cause or discrete vascular lesion. Common precipitants include cardiovascular insults; aortic bypass surgery or aneursymal

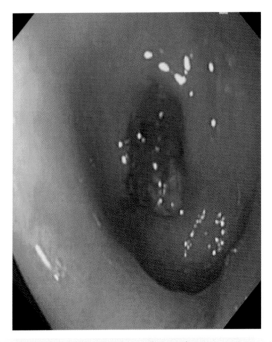

Fig. 1. Stigmata of recent hemorrhage within a diverticulum.

rupture; vasculitis; inherited or acquired hypercoagulable states (eg, pregnancy, oral contraceptives); prolonged, strenuous exercise; and medications or drugs that reduce colonic motility (eg, alosetron) or blood flow (catecholamines). Women with irritable bowel syndrome also appear to be at increased risk [94].

Colonoscopy or flexible sigmoidoscopy have replaced barium enema as the test of choice for colonic ischemia. Endoscopy typically reveals edema, hemorrhage, and ulceration with a sharp line of demarcation between normal and abnormal mucosa (Fig. 2). Histologically, submucosal hemorrhages, intravascular thrombus, and hylanization of the lamina propria are seen, in addition to inflammatory infiltrates. These findings are not pathognomonic, change over time, and may be confused with inflammatory bowel disease and infectious colitis. Most cases of colonic ischemia resolve with conservative treatment. The 15% to 20% of patients who develop gangrene will require surgical intervention and have a substantial risk of death [95]. A minority of patients will develop chronic ischemic colitis or stricture.

Angiodysplasia

Angiodsyplasia are gastrointestinal vascular ectasias, distinct from vascular malformations and telangiectasias seen in other systemic and hereditary disorders. Estimates of angiodysplasia as a source of acute LGIB vary from 2% to 40% [1,9]. Recent data suggests that angiodysplasia are an uncommon source

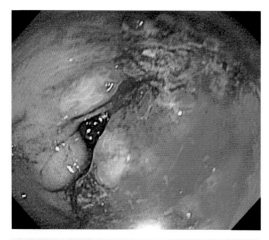

Fig. 2. Colonic ischemia.

of acute LGIB (see Refs. [1,11,96,97]). Angiodysplasia most commonly result in iron deficiency anemia and occult blood loss, and can be found in a small number of asymptomatic individuals [96,97]. Angiodysplasia are thought to be degenerative lesions of the submucosal venules, and are therefore seen predominately in the elderly [98]. A number of comorbid conditions, including valvular heart disease and renal failure have been associated with angiodysplasia. However, these findings were not confirmed in a systematic literature review or a prospective study [99,100].

Overt bleeding from angiodysplasia is typically brisk, painless, and intermittent. Endoscopically angiodsyplasia appear as red, stellate lesions of variable size surrounded by a pale mucosal rim (Fig. 3). The right colon is preferentially involved, although lesions can occur throughout the intestinal tract and are often multiple [101]. Angiography is more sensitive than colonoscopy for detecting angiodysplasia [101]. Bleeding and nonbleeding lesions are characteristically seen as dilated, slowly emptying veins, arterial tufts, or early-filling veins in the arterial phase [102]. Recurrent episodes occur in up to 80% of untreated patients [16]. Fortunately, endoscopic therapy is safe and effective [9].

Postpolypectomy

Clinically relevant bleeding occurs in 1% to 6% of patients undergoing colonoscopic polypectomy [103,104]. Bleeding at the time of polypectomy is amenable to immediate endoscopic hemostasis using various methods. Delayed bleeding typically occurs within 1 week of polypectomy, but can be seen up to 3 weeks following the procedure [104]. Proposed risk factors for postpolypectomy bleeding include large polyps, sessile morphology, and right colon location [105]. The role of aspirin and nonsteroidal anti-inflammatory drugs in postpolypectomy bleeding is controversial. Several large, retrospective studies have found no association [104,106], and current American Society for

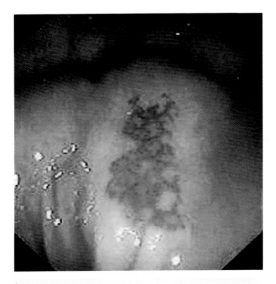

Fig. 3. Angiodysplasia.

Gastrointestinal Endoscopy guidelines state that polypectomy can be performed in patients taking standard doses of these medications [107]. However, the use of anticoagulants, irrespective of the preprocedure international normalized ration (INR), appears to increase the risk of bleeding [106]. Most patients with postpolypectomy bleeding present with mild to moderate blood loss, and many can be managed conservatively [106]. Some patients will have severe hemorrhage requiring emergent intervention and sometimes surgery [104].

Anorectal Sources

Hemorrhoids are the most common anorectal source of acute LGIB and can result in significant hemorrhage. At the time of bleeding, patients often lack other anorectal symptoms, such as pain or pruritis. Anoscopy is superior to flexible endoscopy for detection of hemorrhoids [108]. However, because blood extending beyond the rectal vault can be misleading, endoscopy with retroflexion is also recommended [9]. Most hemorrhoidal bleeding will stop with conservative measures. Patients with significant, refractory hemorrhage may require endoscopic or surgical intervention.

Anorectal fissures, stercoral ulcers, and radiation proctitis are other important anorectal sources of LGIB. Rectal ulcers in particular may result in massive LGIB, and up to 50% are found to have stigmata of recent hemorrhage amenable to endoscopic therapy [109]. Rectal ulcers may be the result of fecal impaction, rectal trauma, or rectal prolapse [109]. Radiation colitis is most often seen in the rectum following radiation therapy for prostate or gynecologic cancer. Radiation colitis typically results in chronic, low-grade bleeding, but can present with more overt blood loss. Scattered or diffuse telangiectasias are seen on endoscopy.

Other Colonic Sources

Cancer and polyps typically result in chronic blood loss and are the source of acute LGIB in only a small percentage of patients. However, neoplasia is among the most important diagnoses to exclude. Similarly, bleeding is a common symptom in inflammatory bowel disease, although it is rarely acute or severe [110]. Certain infectious agents can also result in bloody diarrhea, including *Escherichia coli 0157:H7*, *Salmonella*, *Clostridia difficile*, *Campylobacter*, *Yersinia, and cytomegalovirus*. Rare causes of LGIB include Dieulafuoy's lesions, colonic varices, portal hypertensive enteropathy, Meckel's diverticulum, prostate biopsy sites, and endometriosis.

Small Bowel Sources

Small intestinal sources comprise between 2% and 15% of cases of LGIB [9]. Angiodysplasia are the predominant cause of bleeding from the small intestine followed by lymphoma, erosions/ulcers, and Crohn's disease [111]. Enteroscopy, barium contrast radiography, and capsule endoscopy are appropriate diagnostic modalities. The later technique has begun to revolutionize the diagnosis of bleeding in the small intestine. Patients with small intestinal bleeding require more diagnostic procedures, blood transfusions, and hospital days when compared with patients with UGIB or LGIB [111]. Based on these distinct features and outcomes, Prakash and Zuckerman propose that small intestinal bleeding is a distinct clinical entity [111].

SUMMARY

Lower gastrointestinal bleeding is one of the most common gastrointestinal indications for hospital admission, particularly in the elderly. Diverticulosis accounts for up to 50% of cases, followed by ischemic colitis and anorectal lesions. Though most patients stop bleeding spontaneously and have favorable outcomes, long-term recurrence is a substantial problem for patients with bleeding from diverticulosis and angiodysplasia. The management of LGIB is challenging because of the diverse range of bleeding sources, the large extent of bowel involved, the intermittent nature of bleeding, and the various complicated and often invasive investigative modalities. Advances in endoscopic technology have brought colonoscopy to the forefront of the management of LGIB. However, many questions remained to be answered about its usefulness in routine clinical practice. More randomized controlled trials comparing available diagnostic strategies for LGIB are needed.

References

[1] Longstreth GF. Epidemiology and outcome of patients hospitalized with acute lower gastrointestinal hemorrhage: a population-based study. Am J Gastroenterol 1997;92:419–24.

[2] Longstreth GF. Epidemiology of hospitalization for acute upper gastrointestinal hemorrhage: a population-based study. Am J Gastroenterol 1995;90:206–10.

[3] Kollef MH, O'Brien JD, Zuckerman GR, et al. BLEED: a classification tool to predict outcomes in patients with acute upper and lower gastrointestinal hemorrhage. Crit Care Med 1997;25:1125–32.

[4] Peura DA, Lanza FL, Gostout CJ, et al. The American College of Gastroenterology Bleeding Registry: preliminary findings. Am J Gastroenterol 1997;92:924–8.

[5] Velayos FS, Williamson A, Sousa KH, et al. Early predictors of severe lower gastrointestinal bleeding and adverse outcomes: a prospective study. Clin Gastroenterol Hepatol 2004;2: 485–90.

[6] Al Qahtani AR, Satin R, Stern J, et al. Investigative modalities for massive lower gastrointestinal bleeding. World J Surg 2002;26:620–5.

[7] Chaudhry V, Hyser MJ, Gracias VH, et al. Colonoscopy: the initial test for acute lower gastrointestinal bleeding. Am Surg 1998;64:723–8.

[8] Das A, Ben-Menachem T, Cooper GS, et al. Prediction of outcome in acute lower-gastrointestinal haemorrhage based on an artificial neural network: internal and external validation of a predictive model. Lancet 2003;362:1261–6.

[9] Jensen DM, Machicado GA. Diagnosis and treatment of severe hematochezia. The role of urgent colonoscopy after purge. Gastroenterology 1988;95:1569–74.

[10] Schmulewitz N, Fisher DA, Rockey DC. Early colonoscopy for acute lower GI bleeding predicts shorter hospital stay: a retrospective study of experience in a single center. Gastrointest Endosc 2003;58:841–6.

[11] Strate LL, Orav EJ, Syngal S. Early predictors of severity in acute lower intestinal tract bleeding. Arch Intern Med 2003;163:838–43.

[12] Strate LL, Syngal S. Timing of colonoscopy: impact on length of hospital stay in patients with acute lower intestinal bleeding. Am J Gastroenterol 2003;98:317–22.

[13] Jensen DM, Machicado GA, Jutabha R, et al. Urgent colonoscopy for the diagnosis and treatment of severe diverticular hemorrhage. N Engl J Med 2000;342:78–82.

[14] Painter NS, Burkitt DP. Diverticular disease of the colon: a deficiency disease of Western civilization. BMJ 1971;2:450–4.

[15] Bokhari M, Vernava AM, Ure T, Longo WE. Diverticular hemorrhage in the elderly—is it well tolerated? Dis Colon Rectum 1996;39:191–5.

[16] Boley SJ, DiBiase A, Brandt LJ, et al. Lower intestinal bleeding in the elderly. Am J Surg 1979;137:57–64.

[17] Bloomfeld RS, Rockey DC, Shetzline MA. Endoscopic therapy of acute diverticular hemorrhage. Am J Gastroenterol 2001;96:2367–72.

[18] Browder W, Cerise EJ, Litwin MS. Impact of emergency angiography in massive lower gastrointestinal bleeding. Ann Surg 1986;204:530–6.

[19] Leitman IM, Paull DE, Shires GT III. Evaluation and management of massive lower gastrointestinal hemorrhage. Ann Surg 1989;209:175–80.

[20] Levy R, Barto W, Gani J. Retrospective study of the utility of nuclear scintigraphic-labelled red cell scanning for lower gastrointestinal bleeding. ANZ J Surg 2003;73:205–9.

[21] Suzman MS, Talmor M, Jennis R, et al. Accurate localization and surgical management of active lower gastrointestinal hemorrhage with technetium-labeled erythrocyte scintigraphy. Ann Surg 1996;224:29–36.

[22] Angtuaco TL, Reddy SK, Drapkin S, et al. The utility of urgent colonoscopy in the evaluation of acute lower gastrointestinal tract bleeding: a 2-year experience from a single center. Am J Gastroenterol 2001;96:1782–5.

[23] McGuire HH. Bleeding colonic diverticula. A reappraisal of natural history and management. Ann Surg 1994;220:653–6.

[24] Richter JM, Christensen MR, Kaplan LM, et al. Effectiveness of current technology in the diagnosis and management of lower gastrointestinal hemorrhage. Gastrointest Endosc 1995;41:93–8.

[25] McGuire HH, Haynes BW. Massive hemorrhage for diverticulosis of the colon: guidelines for therapy based on bleeding patterns observed in fifty cases. Ann Surg 1972;175:847–55.

[26] Patel TH, Cordts PR, Abcarian P, et al. Will transcatheter embolotherapy replace surgery in the treatment of gastrointestinal bleeding? Curr Surg 2001;58:323–7.

[27] Thomas S, Wong R, Das A. Economic burden of acute diverticular hemorrhage in the U.S.: a nationwide estimate [abstract W1290]. Presented at the 105th Annual Meeting of the American Gastroenterological Association, New Orleans, 2004.

[28] Comay D, Marshall JK. Resource utilization for acute lower gastrointestinal hemorrhage: the Ontario GI bleed study. Can J Gastroenterol 2002;16:677–82.

[29] Kollef MH, Canfield DA, Zuckerman GR. Triage considerations for patients with acute gastrointestinal hemorrhage admitted to a medical intensive care unit. Crit Care Med 1995;23:1048–54.

[30] Strate L, Saltzman J, Ookubo R, et al. Validation of a clinical prediction rule for severe acute lower intestinal bleeding. Am J Gastroenterol 2005;100:1821–7.

[31] Caos A, Benner KG, Manier J, et al. Colonoscopy after Golytely preparation in acute rectal bleeding. J Clin Gastroenterol 1986;8:46–9.

[32] Brackman MR, Gushchin VV, Smith L, et al. Acute lower gastroenteric bleeding retrospective analysis (the ALGEBRA study): an analysis of the triage, management and outcomes of patients with acute lower gastrointestinal bleeding. Am Surg 2003;69:145–9.

[33] Zuckerman GR, Prakash C. Acute lower intestinal bleeding. Part II: etiology, therapy, and outcomes. Gastrointest Endosc 1999;49:228–38.

[34] Zuckerman GR, Trellis DR, Sherman TM, et al. An objective measure of stool color for differentiating upper from lower gastrointestinal bleeding. Dig Dis Sci 1995;40:1614–21.

[35] Fine KD, Nelson AC, Ellington RT, et al. Comparison of the color of fecal blood with the anatomical location of gastrointestinal bleeding lesions: potential misdiagnosis using only flexible sigmoidoscopy for bright red blood per rectum. Am J Gastroenterol 1999;94:3202–10.

[36] Segal WN, Greenberg PD, Rockey DC, et al. The outpatient evaluation of hematochezia. Am J Gastroenterol 1998;93:179–82.

[37] Graham DJ, Pritchard TJ, Bloom AD. Colonoscopy for intermittent rectal bleeding: impact on patient management. J Surg Res 1993;54:136–9.

[38] Luk GD, Bynum TE, Hendrix TR. Gastric aspiration in localization of gastrointestinal hemorrhage. JAMA 1979;241:576–8.

[39] Cuellar RE, Gavaler JS, Alexander JA, et al. Gastrointestinal tract hemorrhage. The value of a nasogastric aspirate. Arch Intern Med 1990;150:1381–4.

[40] Chalasani N, Clark WS, Wilcox CM. Blood urea nitrogen to creatinine concentration in gastrointestinal bleeding: a reappraisal. Am J Gastroenterol 1997;92:1796–9.

[41] Richards RJ, Donica MB, Grayer D. Can the blood urea nitrogen/creatinine ratio distinguish upper from lower gastrointestinal bleeding? J Clin Gastroenterol 1990;12:500–4.

[42] Snook JA, Holdstock GE, Bamforth J. Value of a simple biochemical ratio in distinguishing upper and lower sites of gastrointestinal haemorrhage. Lancet 1986;1:1064–5.

[43] Jensen DM, Machicado GA. Colonoscopy for diagnosis and treatment of severe lower gastrointestinal bleeding. Routine outcomes and cost analysis. Gastrointest Endosc Clin N Am 1997;7:477–98.

[44] Jiranek GC, Kozarek RA. A cost-effective approach to the patient with peptic ulcer bleeding. Surg Clin North Am 1996;76:83–103.

[45] Lee JG, Turnipseed S, Romano PS, et al. Endoscopy-based triage significantly reduces hospitalization rates and costs of treating upper GI bleeding: a randomized controlled trial. Gastrointest Endosc 1999;50:755–61.

[46] Tada M, Shimizu S, Kawai K. Emergency colonoscopy for the diagnosis of lower intestinal bleeding. Gastroenterol Jpn 1991;26(Suppl 3):121–4.

[47] Colacchio TA, Forde KA, Patsos TJ, et al. Impact of modern diagnostic methods on the management of active rectal bleeding. Ten-year experience. Am J Surg 1982;143:607–10.

[48] Strate LL, Syngal S. Predictors of utilization of early colonoscopy vs. radiography for severe lower intestinal bleeding. Gastrointest Endosc 2005;61:46–52.

[49] Vellacott KD. Early endoscopy for acute lower gastrointestinal haemorrhage. Ann R Coll Surg Engl 1986;68:243–4.

[50] Zuckerman GR, Prakash C. Acute lower intestinal bleeding: part I: clinical presentation and diagnosis. Gastrointest Endosc 1998;48:606–17.

[51] Forde KA. Colonoscopy in acute rectal bleeding. Gastrointest Endosc 1981;27:219–20.

[52] Ponzo F, Zhuang H, Liu FM, et al. Tc-99m sulfur colloid and Tc-99m tagged red blood cell methods are comparable for detecting lower gastrointestinal bleeding in clinical practice. Clin Nucl Med 2002;27:405–9.

[53] Alavi A, Dann RW, Baum S, et al. Scintigraphic detection of acute gastrointestinal bleeding. Radiology 1977;124:753–6.

[54] Alavi A, Ring EJ. Localization of gastrointestinal bleeding: superiority of 99mTc sulfur colloid compared with angiography. AJR Am J Roentgenol 1981;137:741–8.

[55] Gutierrez C, Mariano M, Vander Laan T, et al. The use of technetium-labeled erythrocyte scintigraphy in the evaluation and treatment of lower gastrointestinal hemorrhage. Am Surg 1998;64:989–92.

[56] Hunter JM, Pezim ME. Limited value of technetium 99m-labeled red cell scintigraphy in localization of lower gastrointestinal bleeding. Am J Surg 1990;159:504–6.

[57] Kester RR, Welch JP, Sziklas JP. The 99mTc-labeled RBC scan. A diagnostic method for lower gastrointestinal bleeding. Dis Colon Rectum 1984;27:47–52.

[58] Markisz JA, Front D, Royal HD, et al. An evaluation of 99mTc-labeled red blood cell scintigraphy for the detection and localization of gastrointestinal bleeding sites. Gastroenterology 1982;83:394–8.

[59] Ng DA, Opelka FG, Beck DE, et al. Predictive value of technetium Tc 99m-labeled red blood cell scintigraphy for positive angiogram in massive lower gastrointestinal hemorrhage. Dis Colon Rectum 1997;40:471–7.

[60] Orecchia PM, Hensley EK, McDonald PT, et al. Localization of lower gastrointestinal hemorrhage. Experience with red blood cells labeled in vitro with technetium Tc 99m. Arch Surg 1985;120:621–4.

[61] Rantis PC Jr, Harford FJ, Wagner RH, et al. Technetium-labelled red blood cell scintigraphy: is it useful in acute lower gastrointestinal bleeding? Int J Colorectal Dis 1995;10:210–5.

[62] Voeller GR, Bunch G, Britt LG. Use of technetium-labeled red blood cell scintigraphy in the detection and management of gastrointestinal hemorrhage. Surgery 1991;110:799–804.

[63] Winn M, Weissmann HS, Sprayregen S, et al. The radionuclide detection of lower gastrointestinal bleeding sites. Clin Nucl Med 1983;8:389–95.

[64] Winzelberg GG, Froelich JW, McKusick KA, et al. Scintigraphic detection of gastrointestinal bleeding: a review of current methods. Am J Gastroenterol 1983;78:324–7.

[65] Winzelberg GG, Froelich JW, McKusick KA, et al. Radionuclide localization of lower gastrointestinal hemorrhage. Radiology 1981;139:465–9.

[66] Garofalo TE, Abdu RA. Accuracy and efficacy of nuclear scintigraphy for the detection of gastrointestinal bleeding. Arch Surg 1997;132:196–9.

[67] Gunderman R, Leef JA, Lipton MJ, et al. Diagnostic imaging and the outcome of acute lower gastrointestinal bleeding. Acad Radiol 1998;5(Suppl 2):S303–5.

[68] Bentley DE, Richardson JD. The role of tagged red blood cell imaging in the localization of gastrointestinal bleeding. Arch Surg 1991;126:821–4.

[69] Pennoyer WP, Vignati PV, Cohen JL. Mesenteric angiography for lower gastrointestinal hemorrhage: are there predictors for a positive study? Dis Colon Rectum 1997;40:1014–8.

[70] O'Neill BB, Gosnell JE, Lull RJ, et al. Cinematic nuclear scintigraphy reliably directs surgical intervention for patients with gastrointestinal bleeding. Arch Surg 2000;135:1076–1081 [discussion: 1081–2].

[71] Dusold R, Burke K, Carpentier W, et al. The accuracy of technetium-99m-labeled red cell scintigraphy in localizing gastrointestinal bleeding. Am J Gastroenterol 1994;89:345–8.

[72] Steer ML, Silen W. Diagnostic procedures in gastrointestinal hemorrhage. N Engl J Med 1983;309:646–50.

[73] Browder W, Cerise EJ, Litwin MS. Impact of emergency angiography in massive lower gastrointestinal bleeding. Ann Surg 1986;204:530–6.

[74] Casarella WJ, Galloway SJ, Taxin RN, et al. Lower gastrointestinal tract hemorrhage: new concepts based on arteriography. Am J Roentgenol Radium Ther Nucl Med 1974;121: 357–68.

[75] Cohn SM, Moller BA, Zieg PM, et al. Angiography for preoperative evaluation in patients with lower gastrointestinal bleeding: are the benefits worth the risks? Arch Surg 1998;133:50–5.

[76] Vernava AM, Moore BA, Longo WE, et al. Lower gastrointestinal bleeding. Dis Colon Rectum 1997;40:846–58.

[77] Bloomfeld RS, Smith TP, Schneider AM, et al. Provocative angiography in patients with gastrointestinal hemorrhage of obscure origin. Am J Gastroenterol 2000;95: 2807–12.

[78] Koval G, Benner KG, Rosch J, et al. Aggressive angiographic diagnosis in acute lower gastrointestinal hemorrhage. Dig Dis Sci 1987;32:248–53.

[79] Ryan JM, Key SM, Dumbleton SA, Smith TP. Nonlocalized lower gastrointestinal bleeding: provocative bleeding studies with intraarterial tPA, heparin, and tolazoline. J Vasc Interv Radiol 2001;12:1273–7.

[80] Green B, Rockey D, Portwood G, et al. Urgent colonoscopy for evaluation and management of acute lower gastrointestinal hemorrhage: a randomized controlled study [abstract 140]. Presented at the 104th Annual Meeting of the American Gastroenterological Association, Orlando, FL, 2003.

[81] Tedesco FJ, Waye JD, Raskin JB, et al. Colonoscopic evaluation of rectal bleeding: a study of 304 patients. Ann Intern Med 1978;89:907–9.

[82] Chan FP, Chhor CM. Active lower gastrointestinal hemorrhage diagnosed by magnetic resonance angiography: case report. Abdom Imaging 2003;28:637–9.

[83] Yamaguchi T, Yoshikawa K. Enhanced CT for initial localization of active lower gastrointestinal bleeding. Abdom Imaging 2003;28:634–6.

[84] Pennazio M, Santucci R, Rondonotti E, et al. Outcome of patients with obscure gastrointestinal bleeding after capsule endoscopy: report of 100 consecutive cases. Gastroenterology 2004;126:643–53.

[85] Rastogi A, Schoen RE, Slivka A. Diagnostic yield and clinical outcomes of capsule endoscopy. Gastrointest Endosc 2004;60:959–64.

[86] Adler DG, Knipschield M, Gostout C. A prospective comparison of capsule endoscopy and push enteroscopy in patients with GI bleeding of obscure origin. Gastrointest Endosc 2004;59:492–8.

[87] Ell C, Remke S, May A, et al. The first prospective controlled trial comparing wireless capsule endoscopy with push enteroscopy in chronic gastrointestinal bleeding. Endoscopy 2002;34:685–9.

[88] Costamagna G, Shah SK, Riccioni ME, et al. A prospective trial comparing small bowel radiographs and video capsule endoscopy for suspected small bowel disease. Gastroenterology 2002;123:999–1005.

[89] Ohyama T, Sakurai Y, Ito M, et al. Analysis of urgent colonoscopy for lower gastrointestinal tract bleeding. Digestion 2000;61:189–92.

[90] Painter NS. Diverticular disease of the colon. The first of the Western diseases shown to be due to a deficiency of dietary fibre. S Afr Med J 1982;61:1016–20.

[91] Aldoori WH, Giovannucci EL, Rimm EB, et al. Use of acetaminophen and nonsteroidal anti-inflammatory drugs: a prospective study and the risk of symptomatic diverticular disease in men. Arch Fam Med 1998;7:255–60.

[92] Laine L, Connors LG, Reicin A, et al. Serious lower gastrointestinal clinical events with non-selective NSAID or coxib use. Gastroenterology 2003;124:288–92.

[93] Jun S, Allison JE, Tekawa I, et al. Diverticular bleeding: long term outcome and risk factors for recurrence [abstract W1293]. Presented at the 105th Annual Meeting of the American Gastroenterological Association, 2004.

[94] Walker AM, Bohn RL, Cali C, et al. Risk factors for colon ischemia. Am J Gastroenterol 2004;99:1333–7.

[95] Scharff JR, Longo WE, Vartanian SM, et al. Ischemic colitis: spectrum of disease and outcome. Surgery 2003;134:624–9 [discussion: 629–30].

[96] Foutch PG, Rex DK, Lieberman DA. Prevalence and natural history of colonic angiodysplasia among healthy asymptomatic people. Am J Gastroenterol 1995;90:564–7.

[97] Rockey DC, Koch J, Cello JP, et al. Relative frequency of upper gastrointestinal and colonic lesions in patients with positive fecal occult-blood tests. N Engl J Med 1998;339:153–9.

[98] Boley SJ, Sammartano R, Adams A, et al. On the nature and etiology of vascular ectasias of the colon. Degenerative lesions of aging. Gastroenterology 1977;72:650–60.

[99] Bhutani MS, Gupta SC, Markert RJ, et al. A prospective controlled evaluation of endoscopic detection of angiodysplasia and its association with aortic valve disease. Gastrointest Endosc 1995;42:398–402.

[100] Imperiale TF, Ransohoff DF. Aortic stenosis, idiopathic gastrointestinal bleeding, and angiodysplasia: is there an association? A methodologic critique of the literature. Gastroenterology 1988;95:1670–6.

[101] Richter JM, Hedberg SE, Athanasoulis CA, et al. Angiodysplasia. Clinical presentation and colonoscopic diagnosis. Dig Dis Sci 1984;29:481–5.

[102] Baum S, Athanasoulis CA, Waltman AC, et al. Angiodysplasia of the right colon: a cause of gastrointestinal bleeding. AJR Am J Roentgenol 1977;129:789–94.

[103] Shiffman ML, Farrel MT, Yee YS. Risk of bleeding after endoscopic biopsy or polypectomy in patients taking aspirin or other NSAIDs. Gastrointest Endosc 1994;40:458–62.

[104] Yousfi M, Gostout CJ, Baron TH, et al. Postpolypectomy lower gastrointestinal bleeding: potential role of aspirin. Am J Gastroenterol 2004;99:1785–9.

[105] Sorbi D, Norton I, Conio M, et al. Postpolypectomy lower GI bleeding: descriptive analysis. Gastrointest Endosc 2000;51:690–6.

[106] Hui AJ, Wong RM, Ching JY, et al. Risk of colonoscopic polypectomy bleeding with anticoagulants and antiplatelet agents: analysis of 1657 cases. Gastrointest Endosc 2004;59:44–8.

[107] Eisen GM, Baron TH, Dominitz JA, et al. Guideline on the management of anticoagulation and antiplatelet therapy for endoscopic procedures. Gastrointest Endosc 2002;55:775–9.

[108] Korkis AM, McDougall CJ. Rectal bleeding in patients less than 50 years of age. Dig Dis Sci 1995;40:1520–3.

[109] Kanwal F, Dulai G, Jensen DM, et al. Major stigmata of recent hemorrhage on rectal ulcers in patients with severe hematochezia: Endoscopic diagnosis, treatment, and outcomes. Gastrointest Endosc 2003;57:462–8.

[110] Belaiche J, Louis E. Severe lower gastrointestinal bleeding in Crohn's disease: successful control with infliximab. Am J Gastroenterol 2002;97:3210–1.

[111] Prakash C, Zuckerman GR. Acute small bowel bleeding: a distinct entity with significantly different economic implications compared with GI bleeding from other locations. Gastrointest Endosc 2003;58:330–5.

[112] Wang CY, Won CW, Shieh MJ. Aggressive colonoscopic approaches to lower intestinal bleeding. Gastroenterol Jpn 1991;26(Suppl 3):125–8.

[113] Gutierrez C, Mariano M, Vander Laan T, et al. The use of technetium-labeled erythrocyte scintigraphy in the evaluation and treatment of lower gastrointestinal hemorrhage. Am Surg 1998;64:989–92.

[114] Nicholson ML, Neoptolemos JP, Sharp JF, et al. Localization of lower gastrointestinal bleeding using in vivo technetium-99m-labelled red blood cell scintigraphy. Br J Surg 1989;76:358–61.

Gastroenterol Clin N Am 34 (2005) 665–678

GASTROENTEROLOGY CLINICS
OF NORTH AMERICA

Lower Gastrointestinal Bleeding—Management

Bryan T. Green, MD[a],*, Don C. Rockey, MD[b]

[a]Division of Gastroenterology, Department of Medicine, Duke University Medical Center, Durham, NC 27710, USA
[b]Division of Digestive and Liver Diseases, University of Texas at Southwestern, Dallas, TX, USA

Acute lower gastrointestinal bleeding (LGIB) is distinct clinically from upper gastrointestinal hemorrhage in epidemiology, prognosis, management, and outcome. LGIB encompasses a wide clinical spectrum ranging from trivial hematochezia to massive hemorrhage with shock, requiring emergency hospitalization. The spectrum of LGIB is broad. It may be acute or chronic, obvious or occult. This article focuses on managing patients with acute LGIB. Occult bleeding and obscure bleeding are discussed in articles by Lin and Rockey elsewhere in this issue.

Evaluation of hemodynamic status and resuscitation are the cornerstones in the initial treatment of LGIB. They should take place concomitantly with the history and examination. Postural changes, chest pain, palpitations, syncope, pallor, dyspnea, and tachycardia suggest hemodynamic compromise [1]. An orthostatic decrease in systolic blood pressure of greater than 10 mmHg or an increase in heart rate of more than 10 beats/min indicates an acute loss of at least 15% of blood volume [1,2]. Two large caliber peripheral catheters or a central venous line should be placed immediately in patients with hemodynamic compromise. Initial laboratory studies should include a complete blood count, coagulation profile, type and cross-match, and electrolytes. The use of anticoagulants or nonsteroidal anti-inflammatory drugs (NSAIDs), the presence of liver disease, and serious comorbid medical conditions should be identified rapidly. Coagulopathy or thrombocytopenia should be corrected with fresh frozen plasma or platelet transfusions. In elderly patients or those with a history of cardiac disease, an electrocardiogram or cardiac enzymes should be obtained. The character and frequency of stool output should be noted, as it allows critical assessment of the severity of bleeding. Patients with brown or infrequent stools are unlikely to have brisk bleeding; those with frequent passage of red or maroon stool, however, may have aggressive ongoing bleeding [3].

*Corresponding author. Digestive Diseases Group, 103 Liner Drive, Greenwood, SC 29646.
E-mail address: melissaandbryan@earthlink.net (B.T. Green).

0889-8553/05/$ – see front matter
doi:10.1016/j.gtc.2005.10.001

GENERAL APPROACH

Assessment of Severity in Lower Gastrointestinal Bleeding

In contrast to upper gastrointestinal bleeding, predictors of poor outcome in LGIB are not defined as well [4–7]. Because most episodes of LGIB will stop spontaneously, the early identification of high-risk patients would allow the more selective delivery of urgent therapeutic interventions to the patients most likely to benefit. Two recent studies have examined this. Strate and colleagues [8] retrospectively collected data on 24 clinical variables available in the first 4 hours of evaluation in 252 consecutive patients. They defined severe bleeding as either: continued bleeding within the first 24 hours of hospitalization, or recurrent bleeding after 24 hours of stability. Independent correlates of severe bleeding were: heart rate of at least 100 beats per minute, systolic blood pressure no more than 115 mmHg, syncope, nontender abdominal examination, bleeding per rectum during the first 4 hours of evaluation, aspirin use, and more than two active comorbid medical conditions.

In another study [9] clinical predictors in the first hour of evaluation in patients with severe LGIB included initial hematocrit of no more than 35%, presence of abnormal vital signs 1 hour after initial medical evaluation, and gross blood on initial rectal examination. In this study of 448 prospective patients, severe LGIB was defined as gross red blood per rectum after leaving the emergency department associated with either abnormal vital signs—defined as systolic blood pressure less than 100 mmHg or heart rate above 100 beats per minute—or more than a two-unit blood transfusion during hospitalization. Thus, patients with unstable vital signs, particularly when they persist after initial medical evaluation, are at risk for severe bleeding. Additional studies are needed to refine other predictors.

Evaluation of the Upper Gastrointestinal Tract

An upper gastrointestinal source of bleeding is detected in 10% to 15% of patients presenting with severe hematochezia [10]. Patients with hemodynamic compromise and hematochezia should have a nasogastric tube placed. If bile is present, an upper source is unlikely [11,12]. If the aspirate is nondiagnostic (no blood or bile), or if there is a strong suspicion of an upper bleeding source (ie, history of previous peptic ulcer disease or frequent NSAID use), then an upper endoscopy should be performed before examining the colon [13–15]. An upper endoscopy should be performed if no source of bleeding is identified during colonoscopy.

SPECIFIC INTERVENTIONS/TREATMENTS

Once the patient has been resuscitated, the severity and acuity of bleeding assessed, and an upper gastrointestinal source of bleeding excluded, management rapidly shifts to localization and therapy. The three major modalities available for the treatment of LGIB include: surgery, radiology techniques, and colonoscopy. Pharmacologic measures also are becoming available for a limited number of very specific bleeding sources. The merits of each modality vary by the source of bleeding and the clinical situation.

Colonoscopy

In an effort to improve outcomes by identifying more lesions amendable to endoscopic therapy (either actively bleeding or with stigmata of recent bleeding), interest has increased in performing colonoscopy early in the course of diverticular bleeding. The definition of urgent has varied widely in the literature, from within 8 hours to within 24 hours of presentation [16–21]. Numerous authors have reported urgent colonoscopy to be safe and have a high diagnostic yield in patients who have acute lower gastrointestinal bleeding (Table 1) [17–21]. Bowel preparation generally is recommended before urgent colonoscopy, as complications such as perforation are more common in the uncleansed colon because of decreased visibility. This is usually a polyethylene glycol lavage solution by mouth or nasogastric tube.

In published series, 10% to 15% of patients undergoing urgent colonoscopy received endoscopic therapy (see Table 1). Endoscopic hemostasis methods include injection therapy (epinephrine or saline), heater probe therapy, monopolar and multi-polar electrocoagulation, argon plasma coagulation, hemoclips, and band ligation. In contrast to upper gastrointestinal bleeding, there are no data to compare the effectiveness of each modality in the treatment of diverticular hemorrhage. As a corollary from peptic ulcer bleeding, many experts favor combining epinephrine injection and multi-polar electrocoagulation. Diverticula with active bleeding are injected with 1 mL of epinephrine (dilution, 1:20,000 or 1:10,000) in three or four quadrants around the mouth of the diverticula to stop bleeding. Visible vessels then are treated with multi-polar electrocoagulation with 10 to 15 watts of power with moderate pressure on the vessel [22,23]. Management of adherent clots is more controversial. Some experts recommend cold guillotining of the clot [24]. This involves injecting epinephrine in four quadrants around the pedicle of the clot and shaving it down to 3 to 4 mm above the attachment with a cold polypectomy snare. The underlying stigmata (often a nonbleeding visible vessel) then are treated with multi-polar electrocoagulation. Other experts treat adherent clots by four-quadrant epinephrine injection and then multi-polar electrocoagulation to the base of the clot without intentionally removing it.

Table 1
Urgent colonoscopy for evaluation of lower gastrointestinal bleeding

Study (year)	N	Bowel preparation %	Specific diagnosis N (%)	Endoscopic therapy N (%)
Chaudhry (1998) [17]	85	0	82	17
Kok (1998) [18]	190	85	148	10
Jensen (2000) [19]	121	100	121	10[a]
Angtuaco (2001) [20]	39	100	29	4
Green (2005) [21]	50	100	48	17
Total	485	–	438 (88%)	58 (12%)

[a] Reported only patients who received therapy specifically for diverticular lesions.

Jenson and colleagues [19] employed these hemostasis techniques in the treatment of 10 patients who had either active or stigmata of diverticular hemorrhage. There was a 100% success rate and no early or late rebleeding. Bloomfield and colleagues [25] employed similar hemostasis techniques to 12 patients with diverticular hemorrhage, but one patient experienced early rebleeding, and four had late rebleeding. In a prospective study comparing urgent colonoscopy with angiography-based therapy by Green and colleagues [21], 13 patients who had diverticular hemorrhage were treated with the same endoscopic techniques of epinephrine injection or multi-polar electrocoagulation. Although treatment initially was successful in all patients, two had early rebleeding, and two had late rebleeding. Although the efficacy of epinephrine or multi-polar electrocautery for diverticular hemorrhage has varied, it appears to be safe, as no patients have suffered complications. Numerous case reports and small series also have reported the successful treatment of diverticular hemorrhage with various combinations of epinephrine or multi-polar electrocautery (Fig. 1, Table 2) [17–21,25–32]. Unfortunately, the follow-up has been limited in many of the smaller series.

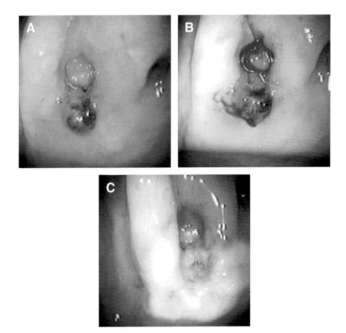

Fig. 1. Treatment of diverticular bleeding—injection and thermal therapy. Shown is a visible vessel associated with a diverticula (A). (B) The lesion after injection with epinephrine (5 cc 1:10,000), and (C) after thermal therapy. (*From* Bloomfeld RS, Rockey DC, Shetzline MA. Endoscopic therapy of acute diverticular hemorrhage. Am J Gastroenterol 2001;96:2369; with permission.)

Table 2
Endoscopic therapy of diverticular hemorrhage with epinephrine and/or contact coagulation

Study (year)	Study type	N	Rebleeding	Treatment
Green (2005) [21]	Prospective	17	4	Epinephrine/coagulation
Jensen (2000) [17]	Prospective	10	0	Epinephrine/coagulation
Bloomfeld (2000) [25]	Retrospective	13	5	Epinephrine/coagulation
Prakash (1999) [32]	Case series	3	0	Coagulation
Ramirez (1996) [27]	Case series	4	0	Epinephrine
Savides (1994) [31]	Case series	3	0	Coagulation
Foutch (1996) [33]	Case series	4	1	Coagulation
Johnston (1986) [26]	Case series	4	0	Coagulation

Innovative therapeutic endoscopists have employed various other techniques to control diverticular hemorrhage [33–35]. Hokama and colleagues [34] described three patients successfully treated with an endoscopic hemoclip, and the clinical experience with hemoclips suggests that this approach is likely to be effective (Fig. 2). Farrell and colleagues [35] described the successful use of endoscopic band ligation to control diverticular hemorrhage in four patients. Although these techniques are exciting, they remain experimental and not ready for widespread application. In contrast, the safety and efficacy of endoscopic hemostasis with epinephrine injection or multi-polar electrocautery are

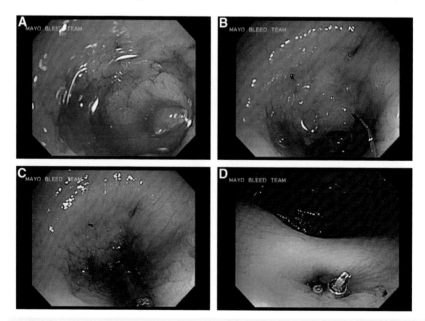

Fig. 2. Treatment of diverticular bleeding—injection and hemoclip therapy. (*A*) Visible vessel inside of a diverticulum. (*B*) After epinephrine injection therapy, the lesion is approached with a hemoclip. (*C*) Lesion is clipped. (*D*) Hemoclip firmly placed on the visible vessel. (*Courtesy of Louis Wang and the Mayo Clinic Bleeding Team.*)

documented and widely available. This should be used when the opportunity arises. Indeed, urgent colonoscopy with endoscopic therapy to actively bleeding diverticula or those with a visible vessel is recommended by the American Society of Gastrointestinal Endoscopy [36].

Angiography

Angiography can identify and localize bleeding accurately, but this requires a bleeding rate of at least 0.5 to 1.0 mL/min to be positive. This sometimes may be a problem because of the intermittent nature of bleeding. It, however, has the advantage of not requiring time to prepare the colon. When the bleeding is identified, it may be treated with intra-arterial infusion of vasopressin or super selective embolization with various agents (gelatin sponge, microcoils, and polyvinyl alcohol particles). Vasopressin was the first modality employed, and it controlled bleeding in up to 91% of cases [37,38]. Unfortunately, the major complication rate was 10% to 20% and included arrhythmias, pulmonary edema, hypertension, and ischemia [39,40]. Rebleeding also occurred in up to 50% of patients after cessation of the infusion [37]. Early attempts at embolization occasionally caused bowel infarction, but current super-selective techniques have made this unusual [39,40]. Selective embolization initially controls hemorrhage in up to 100% of patients, but rebleeding rates are 15% to 40% [39,40]. A recent study by Debaros and colleagues, involving 27 patients undergoing super-selective arterial embolization, found an initial success rate of 100% and a rebleeding rate of only 7% [41]. Another recent study by Burgess and Evans [42] in 15 patients found an initial success rate of 93%, but 53% had rebleeding within 24 hours. Kuo and colleagues [42] achieved immediate hemostasis in 100% of 22 patients, and only 14% experienced rebleeding. A literature review of 144 cases of super-selective arterial embolization found a minor complication rate of 9% and a 0% major complication rate [42]. Although most patients in these studies were bleeding from diverticula, several patients with vascular malformations of the colon and small bowel were included. Because angiographic therapy is felt to be equally effective for both lesions, there is no reason to suspect that this would alter the findings appreciably if diverticular hemorrhage was considered alone.

Surgery

Surgery usually is employed for hemorrhage in two settings: massive or recurrent bleeding. It is required in 15% to 25% of patients who have diverticular bleeding and is recommended for patients with a high transfusion requirement (generally more than four units within a 24-hour period or greater than 10 units total) [43]. Recurrent bleeding from diverticula occurs in 20% to 40% of patients and generally is considered an indication for surgery [44]. In patients with serious comorbid medical conditions and without exsanguinating hemorrhage, this decision should be made carefully. Great effort should be made to accurately localize the site of bleeding preoperatively so that segmental rather than subtotal colectomy can be performed. If the specific bleeding diverticulum can be identified during colonoscopy, the adjacent mucosa should be labeled with India ink so that it can be localized if surgery becomes necessary. Surgical therapy generally is not recommended on the basis of tagged RBC scintigraphy alone, because of variable accuracy of red blood cell (RBC) bleeding scans [45–47]. Tagged RBC scintigraphy is used most often as a screening test before visceral angiography. Although one study [48] showed this policy increased the yield of angiography from 22% to 53%, other studies [49] have had confounding results. The role of RBC scintigraphy in acute LGIB is uncertain and requires further investigation. Whenever possible, it is preferable to perform surgery on an elective basis rather than emergently. Operative mortality is 10% even with accurate localization and up to 57% with blind subtotal colectomy [50–52].

MANAGEMENT OF SPECIFIC CAUSES OF LOWER GASTROINTESTINAL BLEEDING

Diverticula

Diverticula are the most common sourced of acute LGIB (see the article by Strate in this issue). Despite this, there is a paucity of prospective clinical data on specific treatment strategies, and moreover, the ones that are published are primarily case series and small, often nonrandomized studies (see Table 2). The traditional management of diverticular bleeding largely has been supportive, with colonoscopy performed after bleeding had ceased and the colon adequately prepared. Unfortunately, the detection rate of actively or recently bleeding lesions with expectant colonoscopy was low, thus limiting the ability of interventional endoscopic hemostasis to prove benefit. Nonetheless, the available data suggest that endoscopic therapy for diverticular hemorrhage is safe and likely to be beneficial.

It is notable that while in at least 75% of patients, diverticular bleeding stops spontaneously, those in whom it persists or recurs are difficult to manage (and they typically require surgery), and thus, often suffer substantial morbidity and mortality.

Vascular Ectasia

Vascular ectasia most often are located in the right colon. They are found frequently in elderly patients, particularly those with chronic underlying medical conditions, most notably renal failure. Their multi-focal tendency and frequent location in the right colon can make management difficult. Lesions in the colon often present with intermittent hematochezia, while small bowel lesions more often cause occult blood loss and iron deficiency anemia.

Colonoscopy is relatively accurate for identifying vascular ectasias, but unless stigmata of bleeding are found, it is difficult to clearly identify the offending lesion [53]. A poor bowel preparation or the transient decrease in mucosal blood flow associated with narcotic medications used for sedation can make identification difficult [54,55]. Naloxone may enhance their colonoscopic appearance [55]. The best treatment for vascular ectasias is likely therapeutic endoscopy with any of a variety of techniques (ie, electrocoagulation, injection therapy, laser, or argon plasma coagulation) [56]. When multiple lesions are present (and the offending one cannot be ascertained), all should be treated. When contact coagulation is performed on a large angioectasia, the outer margin should be treated first to obliterate feeding vessels and prevent brisk bleeding. Care is needed, because the risk of perforation, especially in the right colon, is significant [57]. Because of this risk, argon plasma coagulation is becoming popular as a noncontact and presumably safer method of treatment [57,58]. Sclerosing agents such as ethanolamine also can be injected, but they are not used widely [59].

Angiography also can identify and treat bleeding from vascular ectasias by intra-arterial vasopressin or embolization techniques [60–62]. Angiography is the treatment of choice for angioectasia in the ileum and jejunum. The intermittent and often obscure nature of bleeding from distal small bowel angioectasia has prompted the use of provocative angiography at some specialty centers. This involves the selective and careful infusion of heparin or thrombolytic agents into the mesenteric vessels supplying the suspected area of bowel in an effort to provoke bleeding from the index lesion, thus allowing therapy [63]. This technique can be employed for bleeding from various sources but requires great expertise and immediate surgical back-up. Hormonal therapy (estrogen) to reduce the frequency of bleeding from multi-focal angioectasia has been studied but was ineffective in recent studies [64,65]. Surgery is rarely necessary, but it is required for uncontrollable or recurrent bleeding. As with diverticular bleeding, surgical outcomes are best when the index lesion has been localized previously to a specific portion of the colon.

Hemorrhoids

Hemorrhoids are common and account for 5% to 10% of acute LGIB, but they rarely cause massive bleeding. Hematochezia should not be ascribed to hemorrhoids without examining the colon. Conservative management with sitz baths, avoidance of straining, and dietary modification are usually effective, although surgical hemorrhoidectomy and rubber band ligation are options for refractory cases [66].

Ischemic Colitis

Ischemic colitis is an increasingly recognized cause of acute lower gastrointestinal hemorrhage. Bleeding is usually mild, diffuse, and infrequently of hemodynamic significance. Treatment is supportive with antibiotics, bowel rest, intravenous fluids, optimization of hemodynamic status, and correction of the precipitating condition [67]. The role of endoscopy is principally to aid in the diagnosis of lesions rather than to treat them. When surgery is necessary, it is most often because of transmural infarction with necrosis rather than bleeding.

Inflammatory and Infectious Colitis

Colitis can be caused by numerous different diseases; each of these is a potential cause of LGIB. Inflammatory bowel disease is the most frequent. Both ulcerative colitis and Crohn's disease can cause severe LGIB [68]. Bleeding is usually self-limited and responds to medical therapy. Infliximab has been used successfully to avert emergency surgery in Crohn's patients who have severe bleeding [69,70]. An endoscopically treatable lesion is uncommon, and surgical intervention may be necessary, especially in patients with recurrent hemorrhage. Patients who have ulcerative colitis are treated best with total colectomy, while patients who have Crohn's disease should have only the diseased segment removed.

Numerous infectious agents can penetrate and injure the colonic mucosa and cause acute LGIB. The principle use of endoscopy is to visualize the mucosa and obtain biopsies to guide the use of antimicrobial agents. Endoscopic therapy with epinephrine injection or multi-polar electrocoagulation is helpful when a precise focus of bleeding is present. In populations with immunosuppression, such as patients who have HIV [71], renal transplant patients [72], or pancreatic transplant patients [73], LGIB often is caused by cytomegalovirus (CMV) ulcers, which often are treated with endoscopic hemostasis followed by medical therapy for CMV.

Radiation Colitis

Radiation therapy to the colon (most commonly the rectum) induces inflammatory changes and can produce radiation colitis. Many different medical

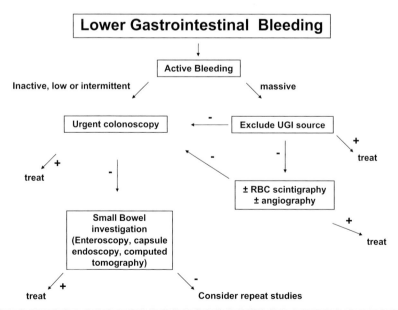

Fig. 3. Management of acute lower gastrointestinal bleeding. One potential algorithm is suggested. In this approach, urgent colonoscopy is advocated. Urgent is taken to mean within 8 hours of presentation. The evidence to support this approach is based on cumulative literature and the author's experience.

therapies, including steroids, hyperbaric oxygen, 5-aminosalicylic acid compounds, and sucralfate have been used to treat radiation proctitis, but little data support their effectiveness [74–76]. Endoscopic therapy with either laser or argon beam coagulation is the most effective treatment [77–81]. A recent study [82] found an 87% success rate with a mean of 2.3 sessions of therapy. Severe complications (severe bleeding, extensive necrosis of the rectum, or perforation) occurred in 10% of patients. Complications can be reduced by using a power setting of less than 45 watts and by treating individual telangiectases rather than diffusely painting the mucosa.

Postpolypectomy Bleeding

Brisk bleeding immediately after polypectomy is usually arterial and can be controlled by resnaring the polyp stalk and holding pressure [83,84]. Delayed bleeding is caused by sloughing of the eschar, and this usually occurs 1 to 2 weeks later. The use of NSAIDS may increase the frequency of this. Delayed bleeding is self-limited in most cases, but persistent bleeding can be treated with various endoscopic techniques. These include injection of epinephrine followed by thermal therapy, loop or band ligation of the remaining polyp stalk, and hemoclips [85–91]. All of these techniques are safe and effective.

SUMMARY

Although acute LGIB is only about one fifth as common and is usually less hemodynamically significant than upper gastrointestinal bleeding, it presents numerous unique clinical challenges. The best diagnostic approach for patients with active bleeding is unknown, but urgent prepared colonoscopy is safe and likely to be beneficial (Fig. 3, Table 2). In patients who have aggressive bleeding or recurrent bleeding, it is critical for the practitioner to judge when angiography and surgery are necessary.

References

[1] Rockey DC. Gastrointestinal bleeding. In: Feldman M, Friedman LS, Sleisenger MH, editors. Sleisenger and Fordra's gastrointestinal and liver disease. 7th edition. Philadelphia: Saunders; 2002. p. 211–48.
[2] Committee on Trauma. American College of Surgeons. Advanced trauma life support. 5th edition. Chicago (IL): American College of Surgeons; 1993. p. 84.
[3] Green BT, Rockey DC. Acute gastrointestinal bleeding. Semin Gastrointest Dis 2003;14: 44–65.
[4] Clason AE, Macleod DA, Elton RA. Clinical factors in the prediction of further haemorrhage or mortality in acute upper gastrointestinal haemorrhage. Br J Surg 1986;73: 985–7.
[5] Provenzale D, Sandler RS, Wood DR, et al. Development of a scoring system to predict mortality from upper gastrointestinal bleeding. Am J Med Sci 1987;294:26–32.
[6] Rockall TA, Logan RF, Devlin HB, et al. Risk assessment after acute upper gastrointestinal haemorrhage. Gut 1996;38:316–31.
[7] Zimmerman J, Siguencia J, Tsvang E, et al. Predictors of mortality in patients admitted to hospital for acute upper gastrointestinal hemorrhage. Scand J Gastroenterol 1995;30:327–31.
[8] Strate LL, Orav EJ, Syngal S. Early predictors of severity in acute lower intestinal tract bleeding. Arch Intern Med 2003;163(7):838–43.

[9] Velayos FS, Williamson A, Sousa KH, et al. Early predictors of severe lower gastrointestinal bleeding and adverse outcomes: a prospective study. Clin Gastroenterol Hepatol 2004;2(6):485–90.

[10] Jensen DM, Machicado GA. Diagnosis and treatment of severe hematochezia: the role of urgent colonoscopy after purge. Gastroenterology 1988;95:1569–74.

[11] Luk GD, Bynum TE, Hendrix TR. Gastric aspiration in localization of gastrointestinal hemorrhage. JAMA 1979;241:576–8.

[12] Cuellar RE, Gavaler JS, Alexander JA, et al. Gastrointestinal tract hemorrhage. The value of a nasogastric aspirate. Arch Intern Med 1990;150:1381–4.

[13] Eisen GM, Dominitz JA, Faigel DO, et al. An annotated algorithmic approach to acute lower gastrointestinal bleeding. Gastrointest Endosc 2001;53:859–63.

[14] Zuccaro G. Management of the adult patient with acute lower gastrointestinal bleeding. Am J Gastroenterol 1998;93:1202–8.

[15] Zuckerman GR, Prakash C. Acute lower intestinal bleeding: part I: clinical presentation and diagnosis. Gastrointest Endosc 1998;48:606–17.

[16] Farrell JJ, Friedman LS. Review article: the management of lower gastrointestinal bleeding. Aliment Pharmacol Ther 2005;21:1281–98.

[17] Chaudhry V, Hyser MJ, Gracias VH, et al. Colonoscopy: the initial test for acute lower gastrointestinal bleeding. Am Surg 1998;64:723–8.

[18] Kok KY, Kum CK, Goh PM. Colonoscopic evaluation of severe hematochezia in an Oriental population. Endoscopy 1998;30:675–80.

[19] Jensen DM, Machicado GA, Jutabha R, et al. Urgent colonoscopy for the diagnosis and treatment of severe diverticular hemorrhage. N Engl J Med 2000;342:78–82.

[20] Angtuaco TL, Reddy SK, Drapkin S, et al. The utility of urgent colonoscopy in the evaluation of acute lower gastrointestinal tract bleeding: a 2-year experience from a single center. Am J Gastroenterol 2001;96(6):1782–5.

[21] Green BT, Rockey DC, Portwood G, et al. Urgent colonoscopy for evaluation and management of acute lower gastrointestinal hemorrhage: a randomized controlled trial. Am J Gastroenterol, in press.

[22] Jenson DM. GI endoscopic hemostasis and tumor treatment- experimental results and techniques. In: Jensen DM, Brunetaud JM, editors. Medical laser endoscopy. Dordrecht (the Netherlands). Kluwer Academic; 1990. p. 45–70.

[23] Jensen DM, Machicado GA. Control of bleeding. In: Raskin JB, Nord HJ, editors. Colonoscopy: principles and techniques. New York: Igaku-Shoin; 1995. p. 317–32.

[24] Jensen DM, Kovacs TOG, Jutabha R, et al. A safe and effective technique for endoscopic removal of adherent clots from GI lesions: cold guillotining after epinephrine injection [abstract]. Gastrointest Endosc 1996;43:297.

[25] Bloomfeld RS, Shetzline M, Rockey D. Urgent colonoscopy for the diagnosis and treatment of severe diverticular hemorrhage. N Engl J Med 2000;342:1608–11.

[26] Johnston JJ, Sones J. Endoscopic heater probe coagulation of the bleeding colonic diverticulum [abstract]. Gastrointest Endosc 1986;84:AB168.

[27] Ramirez FC, Johnson DA, Zierer AT, et al. Successful endoscopic hemostasis of bleeding colonic diverticula with epinephrine injection. Gastrointest Endosc 1996;43:167–70.

[28] Kim Y, Marcon NE. Injection therapy for colonic diverticular bleeding: a case report. J Clin Gastroenterol 1993;17:46–8.

[29] Andress HJ, Mewes A, Lange V. Endoscopic hemostasis of a bleeding diverticulum of the sigma with fibrin sealant. Endoscopy 1993;25:193.

[30] Bertoni G, Conigliaro R, Ricci E, et al. Endoscopic injection hemostasis of colonic diverticular bleeding: a case report. Endoscopy 1990;22:202.

[31] Savides TJ, Jensen DM. Colonoscopic hemostasis for recurrent diverticular hemorrhage associated with a visible vessel: a report of three cases. Gastrointest Endosc 1994;40:70–3.

[32] Prakash C, Chokshi H, Walden DT, et al. Endoscopic hemostasis in acute diverticular bleeding. Endoscopy 1999;31:460–3.

[33] Foutch PG, Zimmerman K. Diverticular bleeding and the pigmented protuberance (sentinel clot): clinical implications, histopathological correlation, and results of endoscopic intervention. Am J Gastroenterol 1996;91:2589–93.

[34] Hokama A, Uehara T, Nakayoshi T, et al. Utility of endoscopic hemoclipping for colonic diverticular bleeding. Gastrointest Endosc 1997;92:543–6.

[35] Farrell JJ, Graeme-Cook F, Kelsey PB. Treatment of bleeding colonic diverticula by endoscopic band ligation: an in-vivo and ex-vivo pilot study. Endoscopy 2003;35:823–9.

[36] Elta GH. Urgent colonoscopy for acute lower GI bleeding. Gastrointest Endosc 2004;59:402–8.

[37] Browder W, Cerise EJ, Litwin MS. Impact of emergency angiography in massive lower gastrointestinal bleeding. Ann Surg 1986;204:530–6.

[38] Clark RA, Colley DP, Eggers FM. Acute arterial gastrointestinal hemorrhage: efficacy of transcatheter control. AJR Am J Roentgenol 1981;136:1185–9.

[39] Ledermann HP, Schoch E, Jost R, et al. Super selective coil embolization in acute gastrointestinal hemorrhage: personal experience in 10 patients and review of the literature. J Vasc Interv Radiol 1998;9:753–60.

[40] Peck DJ, McLoughlin RF, Hughson MN, et al. Percutaneous embolotherapy of lower gastrointestinal hemorrhage. J Vasc Interv Radiol 1998;9:747–51.

[41] DeBarros J, Rosas L, Cohen J, et al. The changing paradigm for the treatment of colonic hemorrhage: super selective angiographic embolization. Dis Colon Rectum 2002;45:802–8.

[42] Kuo WT, Lee DE, Saad WE, et al. Super selective microcoil embolization for the treatment of lower gastrointestinal hemorrhage. J Vasc Interv Radiol 2003;14:1503–9.

[43] Jensen DM, Machicado GA. Colonoscopy for diagnosis and treatment of severe lower gastrointestinal bleeding. Routine outcomes and cost analysis. Gastrointest Endosc Clin N Am 1997;7:477–98.

[44] McGuire HH. Bleeding colonic diverticula. A reappraisal of natural history and management. Ann Surg 1994;220:653–6.

[45] Bloomfeld RS, Rockey DR. Diagnosis and management of lower gastrointestinal bleeding. Curr Opin Gastroenterol 2000;16:89–97.

[46] Voeller GR, Bunch G, Britt LG. Use of technetium-labeled red blood cell scintigraphy in the detection and management of gastrointestinal hemorrhage. Surgery 1991;110:799–804.

[47] Gunderman R, Leef J, Ong K, et al. Scintigraphic screening prior to visceral arteriography in acute lower gastrointestinal bleeding. J Nucl Med 1998;39:1081–3.

[48] Pennoyer WP, Vignati PV, Cohen JL. Mesenteric angiography for lower gastrointestinal hemorrhage: are there predictors for a positive study? Dis Colon Rectum 1997;40:1014–8.

[49] Hyman N, Waye JD. Endoscopic four quadrant tattoo for the identification of colonic lesions at surgery. Gastrointest Endosc 1991;37:56–8.

[50] Bokhari M, Vernava AM, Ure T, et al. Diverticular hemorrhage in the elderly–is it well tolerated? Dis Colon Rectum 1996;39:191–5.

[51] Wagner HE, Stain SC, Gilg M, et al. Systematic assessment of massive bleeding of the lower part of the gastrointestinal tract. Surg Gynecol Obstet 1992;175:445–9.

[52] Parkes BM, Obeid FN, Sorensen VJ, et al. The management of massive lower gastrointestinal bleeding. Am Surg 1993;59:676–8.

[53] Richter JM, Hedberg SE, Athanasoulis CA, et al. Angiodysplasia: clinical presentation and colonoscopic diagnosis. Dig Dis Sci 1984;29:481–5.

[54] Bounds BC, Friedman LS. Lower gastrointestinal bleeding. Gastroenterol Clin N Am 2003;32:1107–25.

[55] Brandt LJ, Spinnell MK. Ability of naloxone to enhance the colonoscopic appearance of normal colon vasculature and colon vascular ectasias. Gastrointest Endosc 1999;49:79–83.

[56] Gupta N, Longo WE, Vernava AM. Angiodysplasia of the lower gastrointestinal tract: an entity readily diagnosed by colonoscopy and primarily managed nonoperatively. Dis Colon Rectum 1995;38:979–82.

[57] Wahab PJ, Mulder CJ, den Hartog G, et al. Argon plasma coagulation in flexible gastrointestinal endoscopy: pilot experiences. Endoscopy 1997;29:176–81.
[58] Johanns W, Luis W, Janssen J, et al. Argon plasma coagulation (APC) in gastroenterology: experimental and clinical experiences. Eur J Gastroenterol Hepatol 1997;9:581–7.
[59] Bemvenuti GA, Julich MM. Ethanolamine injection for sclerotherapy of angiodysplasia of the colon. Endoscopy 1998;30:564–9.
[60] Evangelista PT, Hallisey MJ. Transcatheter embolization for acute lower gastrointestinal hemorrhage. J Vasc Interv Radiol 2000;11:601–6.
[61] Zuckerman GR, Prakash C. Acute lower intestinal bleeding. Part II: etiology, therapy, and outcomes. Gastrointest Endosc 1999;49:228–38.
[62] DeBarros J, Rosas L, Cohen J, et al. The changing paradigm for the treatment of colonic hemorrhage: super selective angiographic embolization. Dis Colon Rectum 2002;45: 802–8.
[63] Shetzline MA, Suhocki P, Dash R, et al. Provocative angiography in obscure gastrointestinal bleeding. South Med J 2000;93(12):1205–8.
[64] Lewis BS, Salomon P, Rivera-MacMurray S, et al. Does hormonal therapy have any benefit for bleeding angiodysplasia? J Clin Gastroenterol 1992;15:99–103.
[65] Barkin JS, Ross BS. Medical therapy for chronic gastrointestinal bleeding of obscure origin. Am J Gastroenterol 1998;93:1250–4.
[66] Randall GM, Jensen DM, Machicado GA, et al. Prospective randomized comparative study of bipolar versus direct current electrocoagulation for treatment of bleeding internal hemorrhoids. Gastrointest Endosc 1994;40:403–10.
[67] Green BT, Tendler DA. Ischemic colitis: a clinical review. South Med J 2005;98:217–22.
[68] Pardi DS, Loftus EV, Tremaine WJ, et al. Acute major gastrointestinal hemorrhage in inflammatory bowel disease. Gastrointest Endosc 1999;49:153–7.
[69] Tsujikawa T, Nezu R, Andoh A, et al. Infliximab as a possible treatment for the hemorrhagic type of Crohn's disease. J Gastroenterol 2004;39(3):284–7.
[70] Papi C, Gili L, Tarquini M, et al. Infliximab for severe recurrent Crohn's disease presenting with massive gastrointestinal hemorrhage. J Clin Gastroenterol 2003;36(3):238–41.
[71] Bini EJ, Weinshel EH, Falkenstein DB. Risk factors for recurrent bleeding and mortality in human immunodeficiency virus infected patients with acute lower GI hemorrhage. Gastrointest Endosc 1999;49:748–53.
[72] Stylianos S, Forde KA, Benvenisty AI, et al. Lower gastrointestinal hemorrhage in renal transplant recipients. Arch Surg 1988;123:739–44.
[73] Green BT, Tuttle-Newhall J, Suhocki P, et al. Massive gastrointestinal hemorrhage due to rupture of a donor pancreatic artery pseudoaneurysm in a pancreas transplant patient. Clin Transplant 2004;18(1):108–11.
[74] Kochhar R, Sharma SC, Gupta BB, et al. Rectal sucralfate in radiation proctitis. Lancet 1988;2:400.
[75] Sasai T, Hiraishi H, Suzuki Y, et al. Treatment of chronic post-radiation proctitis with oral administration of sucralfate. Am J Gastroenterol 1998;93:1593–5.
[76] Stockdale AD, Biswas A. Long-term control of radiation proctitis following treatment with sucralfate enemas. Br J Surg 1997;84:379.
[77] Lee J. Radiation proctitis—a niche for the argon plasma coagulator. Gastrointest Endosc 2002;56:779–81.
[78] Denton AS, Andreyev HJ, Forbes A, et al. Systematic review for nonsurgical interventions for the management of late radiation proctitis. Br J Cancer 2002;87:134–43.
[79] Taieb S, Rolachon A, Cenni JC, et al. Effective use of argon plasma coagulation in the treatment of severe radiation proctitis. Dis Colon Rectum 2001;44:1766–71.
[80] Viggiano TR, Zighelboim J, Ahlquist DA, et al. Endoscopic Nd:YAG laser coagulation of bleeding from radiation proctopathy. Gastrointest Endosc 1993;39:513–7.
[81] Taylor JG, Disario JA, Bjorkman DJ. KTP laser therapy for bleeding from chronic radiation proctopathy. Gastrointest Endosc 2000;52:353–7.

[82] Canard JM, Vedrenne B, Bors G, et al. Long-term results of treatment of hemorrhagic radiation proctitis by argon plasma coagulation. Gastroenterol Clin Biol 2003;27(5):455–9.

[83] Waye JD, Kahn O, Auerbach ME. Complications of colonoscopy and flexible sigmoidoscopy. Gastrointest Endosc Clin N Am 1996;6:343–77.

[84] Rex DK, Lewis BS, Waye JD. Colonoscopy and endoscopic therapy for delayed postpolypectomy hemorrhage. Gastrointest Endosc 1992;38:127–9.

[85] Sobrino-Faya M, Martinez S, Gomez Balado M, et al. Clips for the prevention and treatment of postpolypectomy bleeding (hemoclips in polypectomy). Rev Esp Enferm Dig 2002;94: 457–62.

[86] Brooker JC, Saunders BP, Shah SG, et al. Treatment with argon plasma coagulation reduces recurrence after piecemeal resection of large sessile colonic polyps: a randomized trial and recommendations. Gastrointest Endosc 2002;55:371–5.

[87] Parra-Blanco A, Kaminaga N, Kojima T, et al. Hem clipping for postpolypectomy and postbiopsy colonic bleeding. Gastrointest Endosc 2000;51:37–41.

[88] Ardengh JC, Ferrari AP, Ganc AJ, et al. Endoscopic banding ligation and postpolypectomy bleeding. Endoscopy 1999;31:S61.

[89] Dumonceau JM, Deviere J. Early rebleeding after successful hem clipping of a postpolypectomy rectal ulcer. Endoscopy 1999;31:S54–5.

[90] Uno Y, Satoh K, Tuji K, Wada T, et al. Endoscopic ligation by means of clip and detachable snare for management of colonic postpolypectomy hemorrhage. Gastrointest Endosc 1999;49:113–5.

[91] Waye JD. Management of complications of colonoscopic polypectomy. Gastroenterologist 1993;1:158–64.

Gastroenterol Clin N Am 34 (2005) 679–698

GASTROENTEROLOGY CLINICS
OF NORTH AMERICA

Obscure Gastrointestinal Bleeding

Sauyu Lin, MD[a], Don C. Rockey, MD[b],*

[a]Division of Gastroenterology, Duke University Medical Center, Durham, NC, USA
[b]Division of Digestive and Liver Diseases, University of Texas Southwestern Medical Center, 5323 Harry Hines Boulevard, Dallas, TX 75390–8887, USA

Obscure gastrointestinal (GI) bleeding is generally accepted to be GI bleeding that persists or recurs without an obvious etiology after standard endoscopic examination (routine upper endoscopy and colonoscopy) [1]. Obscure GI bleeding may be categorized into two groups: obscure occult and obscure overt bleeding. Obscure occult GI bleeding is defined as persistently positive fecal occult blood testing with or without iron deficiency and without frank blood loss recognizable to the patient or the physician. Obscure overt GI bleeding is defined as clinically evident bleeding that persists or recurs after negative endoscopic examinations. This article covers the latter form of bleeding. GI bleeding leads to more than 300,000 hospitalizations per year. The cause of bleeding in most of these patients is defined by routine endoscopic and radiographic techniques. Approximately 10% to 20% of these patients, however, do not have an identified bleeding source. Fortunately, only half of these patients do not have a recurrent bleeding event. A small proportion (approximately 5% overall) of these patients have recurrent bleeding of unclear etiology, however, leading to extensive and repetitive testing [2,3].

Reasons leading to a missed diagnosis include lesions that have stopped bleeding during endoscopic examination and are overlooked; significant anemia and volume contraction causing lesions to look less obvious; very slow bleeding or intermittent bleeding leading to negative endoscopic and nuclear scans; and, importantly, lesions in the small bowel that are not detected by routine examinations [4]. Investigation of the small bowel is problematic for several reasons. First, the length of small bowel (average 6.7 m) makes its complete visualization difficult. The free intraperitoneal location and active contractility of the small bowel makes endoscope passage difficult. Finally, the multiple overlying loops of the small bowel makes contrast studies less than optimal [5].

The source of obscure GI bleeding may be attributable to any of a number of different etiologies (Box 1). The age of the patient is a very important factor in the differential diagnosis of obscure GI bleeding [4]. Patients who are younger than 40 are more likely to suffer from small bowel tumors, such as lymphomas,

*Corresponding author. E-mail address: don.rockey@utsouthwestern.edu (D.C. Rockey).

0889-8553/05/$ – see front matter
doi:10.1016/j.gtc.2005.08.005
gastro.theclinics.com

Box 1: Differential diagnosis of obscure gastrointestinal bleeding[a]

Mass lesions
  Carcinoma (any type)
  Large (>1.5 cm) adenoma (any site)

Inflammation
  Ulcer (any site)[b]
  Cameron lesions
  Idiopathic cecal ulcer

Vascular
  Vascular ectasia (any site)[b]
  Watermelon stomach
  Hemangioma

Other
  Diverticula

Potential lesions leading to all forms of occult GI bleeding are shown.

[a]See list on following page for less frequent, but difficult to recognize, causes of obscure bleeding.
[b]Most common abnormalities, typically located in the small bowel.

carcinoids, and adenocarcinomas; Meckel's diverticulum; Dieulafoy lesion; polyps from a hereditary polyposis syndrome, such as familial polyposis syndrome; or Crohn's disease. Patients who are older than 40 are more prone to bleeding from vascular lesions, which may comprise up to 40% of all causes; nonsteroidal anti-inflammatory drug–induced ulcers; Cameron erosions; and other less common etiologies, such as aortoenteric fistulas in patients with prior aortic aneurysm repair, hemosuccus pancreaticus in patients with necrotizing pancreatitis or pancreatic transplantation, or hemobilia in patients with hepatocellular malignancy, recent liver biopsy, or trauma [6].

APPROACH TO EVALUATION OF THE OBSCURE BLEEDER

The evaluation of obscure GI bleeding usually begins with a history of symptoms, past medical history, medications, family history, and a physical examination, although a history may not always be helpful in suggesting a diagnosis. Careful attention should be focused on the small bowel with reference to weight loss and obstructive symptoms. Elderly patients, patients with a history of renal disease, a connective tissue disease, or von Willebrand's disease may be at higher risk for vascular lesions. Surgical patients may be at higher risk for anastomotic bleeds or aortoenteric fistulas. Users of nonsteroidal anti-inflammatory drugs have an increased risk of small bowel ulcerations. Important family history includes a history of inflammatory bowel disease, malignancies, or hereditary telangiectasias. Additionally, history and physical examination should focus on elements likely to be active in patients with easily overlooked lesions. Difficult-to-identify causes of obscure GI bleeding include the following:

Hemosuccus pancreaticus
Hemobilia
Aortoenteric fistula
Dieulafoy's ulcer (stomach more than other sites)
Meckel's diverticulum
Extraesophageal varices (gastric, small bowel, colonic)

A key first step in the evaluation is typically to localize the site (ie, upper or lower GI tract) of bleeding. Patients who suffer from hematemesis usually have a lesion proximal to the ligament of Treitz. The appearance of the stool, which is largely dependent on blood transit time, may also be suggestive of location of the bleeding. Blood that has been in the GI tract for less than 5 hours is usually red, whereas blood present for more than 20 hours is usually melenic. Upper GI, small bowel, or a slow right colon bleeding usually produces melena, whereas patients with hematochezia typically have left colonic or rectal lesions [7]. Although melena and hematochezia are typically associated with upper and lower GI tract bleeding, respectively, it should be emphasized that patients with slow oozing from the distal small bowel or cecum may have melena and occasional patients with aggressive bleeding from an upper GI source may present with hematochezia.

A proposed approach to patients with obscure bleeding is presented in Fig. 1. In general, in patients with recurrent obscure bleeding, repeat endoscopy directed at the most likely site of bleeding is usually warranted at least one additional time after the index endoscopy. It has been well documented in the literature that re-examination of the upper GI tract within reach of a standard gastroscope (or an enteroscope) identifies lesions in a substantial proportion of patients [8–10]. Familiarity, however, with uncommon or subtle bleeding lesions is required [11]. If a lesion cannot be identified, further evaluation depends on the briskness of bleeding. In those with active bleeding, technetium-99 radionuclide scanning or angiography should be performed. Unfortunately, this approach allows only confirmation of the site of bleeding. Angiography is less sensitive than technetium-99 radionuclide scanning but may allow treatment [12]. In some patients, diagnostic tests, such as CT or Meckel's scan, may be helpful. In patients with subacute or intermittent bleeding in whom repeat endoscopy of the upper or lower GI tract is negative, the focus of investigation should rapidly move to the small intestine. The lesions most commonly identified in the small bowel include tumors and vascular ectasias, which vary in frequency depending on age. In patients between 30 and 50, tumors are the most common abnormalities (in patients less than 25 years of age, Meckel's diverticula are the most common

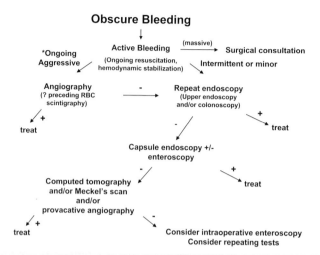

Fig. 1. Algorithm for management of obscure GI bleeding. The management of individual patients varies greatly depending on specific patient features and local expertise. The algorithm shown is based on the available literature and the authors' experience. Patients with active bleeding should undergo repeat endoscopy or a localization procedure. In those with aggressive bleeding, angiography is likely to reveal a source, and specific therapy may be possible. Endoscopy is generally indicated in others, with the exception of those having undergone many endoscopic procedures (and in whom the endoscopy was unhelpful). Evaluation then shifts to the small bowel, and may be with capsule endoscopy, enteroscopy, or both. Special studies, such as CT–Meckel's scanning, are indicated in specific circumstances. Intraoperative enteroscopy is reserved for patients with refractory bleeding and negative studies, and requires a specialized team approach.

source of small bowel bleeding), whereas vascular ectasias predominate in the elderly [13].

Small bowel examination can be performed with a number of radiologic and endoscopic modalities. These can be divided into radiographic, endoscopic, and surgical modalities. Radiographic techniques include barium studies, such as small bowel follow-through (SBFT) and enteroclysis; nuclear studies, such as tagged red blood cell scans and Meckel's scan; cross-section imaging, such as CT and MRI; and angiography. Endoscopic techniques include standard endoscopy, small bowel endoscopy, and capsule endoscopy. Surgical procedures include exploratory laparotomy with and without endoscopic assistance. Each of these modalities is reviewed next.

PRIMARY DIAGNOSTIC MODALITIES IN OBSCURE BLEEDING
Radiographic Modalities
Small bowel follow-through
SBFT is often used for the evaluation of obscure GI blood loss [14,15]. The use of SBFT for this indication, however, seems to be questionable. The diagnostic yield of SBFT may be as low as 0% [16]. A high false-negative rate has also

been reported [17,18]. In a large case series, Rabe and coworkers [15] found a probable diagnosis in only 12 (5.6%) of 215 patients. The most common finding was small bowel diverticulosis, followed by small bowel tumors and Crohn's disease. Although small bowel diverticuli may lead to GI bleeding, it is controversial whether their presence definitively defines a bleeding source. For patients with a high index of suspicion for the presence of small bowel disease, such as small bowel malignancy or Crohn's disease, the diagnostic yield may be higher. Kusumoto and coworkers [19] found that SBFT detected 83% of small bowel tumors. In patients with suspected Crohn's disease, SBFT may have a sensitivity of >90% [20–22]. Notwithstanding, available data suggest that unless malignancy or Crohn's disease is suspected, SBFT has little use in the evaluation of obscure GI bleeding.

Enteroclysis

Enteroclysis is a modified form of SBFT that seems to be superior to SBFT for examination of the small bowel. A 10F catheter tube is placed in the distal duodenum or proximal jejunum using fluoroscopy. A double-contrast solution consisting of barium and air, water, or methylcellulose is then infused under high pressure (usually on the order of 75 mL per minute). This rapid rate of infusion allows better distention and visualization of the small bowel. The diagnostic yield in patients with obscure GI bleeding seems to be superior to SBFT, with results varying from 10% to 21% [23–25]. Small bowel tumors seem to be the most common diagnosis, followed by Meckel's diverticulum and Crohn's disease of the terminal ileum [24,25]. Enteroclysis is particularly useful in patients with obscure bleeding believed to be secondary to small bowel malignancy or Crohn's disease. Compared with SBFT, the sensitivity of enteroclysis was 95% compared with 61% for small bowel cancers [26]. In patients suspected of suffering from Crohn's disease, sensitivity has been estimated to be as high as 93% to 100% and specificity 97% to 99% [27]. Several studies have suggested that enteroclysis is superior to SBFT for this indication [27–29]; however, a prospective study found comparable results and suggested SBFT may be preferable because of better patient tolerance and superior examination of gastroduodenal disease (see Table 1). This is still highly debated [20,30–33]. With the advent of capsule endoscopy, however, the use of SBFT or enteroclysis for obscure GI bleeding has declined substantially.

Technetium-labeled nuclear scans

Because of their mode of action, bleeding scans are only useful in the setting of active GI bleeding. Two types of nuclear scans may be used in this setting: the technetium 99m-labeled red blood cell scan and the technetium 99m-labeled sulfur colloid scan. The tagged red blood cell scan is more commonly applied. It can reportedly detect active bleeding at a rate of 0.10 mL/min [2]. During this scan, 20 mL of red blood cells are tagged with technetium and subsequently reinjected into the patient. In general, images are taken every 3 seconds for the first minute, every 5 minutes for the next 45 minutes, and then every 15

Table 1
Studies in obscure gastrointestinal bleeding

Study	Therapy (Y/N)	Advantages	Disadvantages
SBFT	N	Safe	Insensitive
Enteroclysis	N	Safe	Poor for mucosal lesions
Scintigraphy	N	Safe	Localization only
Angiography	Y	Often helpful in active bleeding	Unable to identify lesion, invasive
CT	N	Safe	Little experience
Enteroscopy	Y	Wide experience	Unclear outcome data
Capsule endoscopy	N	Safe	Unclear outcome data
Surgery	Y	Great potential for therapeutic efficacy	Highly invasive

Abbreviation: SBFT, small bowel follow-through.

to 60 minutes depending on the clinical setting. During the sulfur colloid scan, 20 mL of blood is again tagged and reinjected. The sulfur colloid scan is extremely sensitive, with a reported ability to detect bleeding as slow as 0.05 mL/min. There is intense reuptake, however, in the reticuloendothelial system. The scan can only be performed every 1 minute for the first 10 minutes. After this time period, uptake in the liver and spleen limits further visualization, especially of the upper GI tract and hepatic and splenic flexures. The diagnostic yield of nuclear scanning in patients with obscure GI bleeding has been estimated to be between 15% and 70% in patients with overt obscure GI bleeding [34–39]. The heterogeneity of studies, however, makes the true diagnostic yield difficult to discern. The sensitivity for active bleeding has been reported to be good, with reports of greater than 90%, superior to that of angiography [35,37]. The positive predicative value has also been reported to be as high as 84%; however, a false localization rate of 59% has also been reported [36–38,40]. In addition, when definitive lesions are verified by other means, the accuracy of a positive scan for lesion localization may be as poor as 41% [40,41]. Voeller and coworkers [38] evaluated 85 patients with proved bleeding sites by arteriography, endoscopy, or surgery, and found that scintigraphy failed to localize a bleeding site in 85% of patients. The yield seems to be higher if an immediate scan blush is seen (61%) compared with when a late blush is present (7%) [42]. In the setting of a negative tagged red blood cell scan, repeating a scan 12 to 24 hours after injection may be useful if the patient rebleeds; however, it may also be misleading and identify areas of blood that has pooled and not the primary site of bleeding [1]. In patients with obscure GI bleeding, there are several drawbacks to nuclear scanning. First, nuclear scanning localizes active bleeding to a region of the abdomen, not a specific site; even a positive scan cannot provide an etiology for the bleeding [34]. In addition, because scanning is not therapeutic, a follow-up study, such as arteriogram or endoscopic examination, must be subsequently performed. Nuclear scanning probably should be reserved for patients suffering from bleeding believed to be inaccessible by endoscopy and at centers with angiographic capabilities.

Meckel's scan

A Meckel's diverticulum is a vestige of the omphalomesenteric duct, and is the most common congenital GI anomaly. It is commonly located several centimeters proximal to the ileocecal valve and often contains heterotopic gastric mucosa that becomes ulcerated and bleeds [43,44]. It is the cause of nearly 50% of GI bleeding in patients younger than 3 years of age [45]. The Meckel's scan uses technetium pertechnetate tracer because of the tracer's affinity to accumulate in gastric mucosa. The test is quite useful in the pediatric population, with sensitivity as high as 81% to 90% [46,47]. False-negative scans have been reported, and repeat scans have been found to be useful [48]. Unfortunately, the sensitivity of the scan is much lower in the adult population, estimated to be approximately 62% [45,49]. This low yield is attributable to insufficient gastric mucosa in the diverticulum. Patients who have lived to adulthood without a prior history of bleeding are suspected of having less ectopic gastric mucosa in the diverticulum, because higher concentrations lead to GI bleeding earlier in life. In addition, pooling of tracer in the bladder may lead to false-negative studies [45]. Several modifications to the test may improve the diagnostic yield in the adult population. The addition of pentagastrin, which increases acid production from parietal cells, may increase the diagnostic yield [50,51]. Histamine blockers may lead to longer retention within the gastric mucosa and a higher likelihood of a positive scan. Saline lavage of the stomach and bladder before scanning may decrease false-negatives and -positives [49,50,52–54]. A modification of the standard Meckel's scan using single-photon emission CT has been shown to detect heterotopic gastric mucosa [55]. The Meckel's scan seems to be very useful in the pediatric population, but its role in adults with obscure GI bleeding is still not well defined.

Angiography

Angiography may be a useful diagnostic and therapeutic tool in patients who are actively (and more aggressively) bleeding (see also the article by Miller and Smith elsewhere in this issue). Angiography is less sensitive than nuclear scintigraphy, is invasive, and is rarely used as first-line evaluation. It is often performed after a positive nuclear scan or failed therapeutic endoscopy [56]. Angiography can demonstrate extravasation of contrast if bleeding is faster than 0.5 mL/min, although 1 mL/min is optimal [57]. In addition, it can also identify nonbleeding lesions by its vascular pattern, such as vascular ectasias [58]. Venous bleeding is not identified. The diagnostic yield of angiography in patients with obscure GI bleeding is approximately 40%, although yields as high as 80% have been reported [12,59,60]. It seems to be most sensitive when performed shortly after an early positive tagged red blood cell scan [42]. Alternatively, angiography has been especially useful in patients presenting with postoperative GI hemorrhage [61]. It is important to emphasize that significant complications have been associated with angiography and include renal failure, arterial dissection, and ischemic colitis, reported in up to 11% of patients [62].

Once a lesion has been identified, interventional angiography with intra-arterial vasopressin or embolization can be implemented therapeutically (see the article by Miller and Smith elsewhere in this issue). Initial cessation of bleeding occurs in 70% to 90% of patients with obscure GI bleeding [63–66]. Complications, such as bowel infarction, may occur in up to 10% of cases [66].

If standard angiography is negative, provocative angiography may be considered. In this type of study, anticoagulants, vasodilators, and thrombolytics, such as heparin, tolazoline, tissue plasminogen activator, and urokinase, have all been used to induce bleeding [67–71]. The success of provocative angiography is unclear (see the article by Miller and Smith elsewhere in this issue), and the use of provocative angiography should be reserved for select patients at academic centers with well-trained interventional radiologists.

Angiography seems to be useful in patients with early positive nuclear scans, in postoperative patients, and in patients with severe bleeding not diagnosed or unable to be treated by endoscopy. It may also be helpful in detecting otherwise undiagnosed vascular lesions. Complications can occur, however, and it must be undertaken in a carefully controlled environment with skilled interventionalists (see the article by Miller and Smith elsewhere in this issue). It is generally reserved for specific situations in which other modalities have failed.

CT

Helical CT angiogram is a modified form of angiography. Thirty seconds after contrast is injected into the abdominal aorta, a rapid-acquisition CT scan is performed with 10-mm slices 5 mm apart. Active bleeding is seen as extravasation of contrast medium into the intestinal lumen. Bleeding rates over 6 mL/min are believed to be necessary for an aortogram to be diagnostic, whereas selective angiography requires a much lower bleeding rate of 0.5 mL/min [72]. Only one study evaluating the use of helical CT angiography in obscure GI bleeding has been performed. In this study, in which 18 patients with obscure GI bleeding were examined using both helical CT angiogram and conventional angiogram, evidence of hemorrhage was found in 13 (72%) of 18 patients using helical CT, two more than angiogram alone [72]. This suggested that helical CT angiogram might be more sensitive than angiogram alone in detecting slower GI bleeds. Further study, however, is needed. In addition, helical CT angiography may also be useful in the evaluation of colonic vascular lesions, with a sensitivity of 70% and specificity of 100% compared with colonoscopy and conventional angiography [73]. Because of the invasive nature of helical CT angiogram, helical CT alone may be preferred. In a swine model of GI bleeding, contrast extravasation using contrast-enhanced blood at 0.3 to 1 mL/min was performed over a 30-second period followed by unopacified blood during helical CT imaging. It seemed that helical CT has the potential to detect rates of hemorrhage of 0.5 mL/min or less [74,75]. In a case report by Miller and coworkers [76,77], a patient with obscure GI bleeding received a helical CT scan after drinking 1 L of water as a negative contrast agent. Intravenous contrast was then injected at a rate of 5 mL/s and postcontrast scans obtained during the arterial and venous phase at 6.5-mm slice thickness reconstructed at 3-mm intervals. A focus of bleeding was identified in the jejunum on the arterial phase. In the operating room, partial jejunal resection revealed submucosa hemorrhage from cholesterol thrombi. Using a three-phase helical CT (unenhanced, arterial [30-second delay], delayed [2 minute]) scan, Ernst and coworkers [78] evaluated 24 patients with acute GI bleeding. Of these patients, 19 had confirmed sources of bleeding using colonoscopy, push enteroscopy, or surgery. Helical CT detected 15 (79%) of 19 sources. Although still undergoing study, helical CT seems to be a promising, noninvasive diagnostic tool in the evaluation of obscure GI bleeding.

MRI

No studies have evaluated the use of MRI in obscure GI bleeding. MRI may visualize changes, such as mucosal thickening, stricturing, and ulcerations, to suggest evidence of Crohn's disease and small bowel tumors. Because of limited spatial resolution, lesions have also been missed [79]. No formal comparison between MRI and other modalities, such as CT and barium studies, has been performed for this etiology. Currently, there is no role for the use of MRI in the evaluation of obscure GI bleeding.

Endoscopic Modalities

Routine endoscopy

In patients with a negative upper endoscopy and colonoscopy, the use of repeating the upper endoscopic examination has a surprisingly high yield, ranging from 25% to 64% [8,10,80,81]. Commonly missed lesions include vascular ectasias, polyps, Cameron ulcers, and peptic ulcers. Repeating a colonoscopy seems to be less useful, with a diagnostic yield of only 6% [2]. Thus, in patients with obscure GI bleeding, a repeat upper endoscopy should always be performed. The yield of random small bowel biopsies in patients with occult GI bleeding and iron deficiency anemia for celiac disease may be as high as 12% [82,83]. The use of random small bowel biopsies and a repeat colonoscopy are more controversial and should be performed on a case-by-case basis.

Enteroscopy

Small bowel enteroscopy (SBE) is currently the best endoscopic modality to investigate the small bowel, and this tool has become a cornerstone in the management of patients with obscure GI bleeding [84]. Introduced by Ogoshi and coworkers [85] in 1973, SBE became more widely used after Parker and Agayoff [86] used a colonoscope for successful visualization of the jejunum. With the development of longer instruments in combination with video technology, the use of SBE in the evaluation of obscure GI bleeding has become routine. Previously used with an overtube, studies have suggested that the use of the overtube may increase intubation into the jejunum but does not improve diagnostic yield and may increase complication rates [87–91]; the overtube is now rarely used. The diagnostic yield for SBE varies between 13% and 78% [8,10, 17,80,81,92–97]. The most common findings include small bowel vascular lesions followed by ulcerations and malignancies [8,80,81]. Although treatment of lesions found on enteroscopy, especially vascular lesions, may decrease hospitalizations and transfusion requirements, up to 31% of all patients who undergo push enteroscopy for evaluation and treatment of obscure GI bleeding continue to rebleed over time [92,98].

Unfortunately, SBE can only examine a relatively short portion of the small bowel, estimated to be between 50 and 150 cm distal to the pylorus; however, even under fluoroscopy, the true depth of insertion is unreliable [87,93,94,98]. Most recently, the use of double balloon enteroscopy has gained attention as a method of deeper intubation of the small bowel. Initially introduced by Yamamoto in 2001, the double balloon enteroscope consists of a working length of 200 cm, a flexible overtube with a length of 140 cm, and latex balloons attached to the tip of the enteroscope and the overtube [99–102]. In a preliminary report, the diagnostic yield of double balloon enteroscopy in those with obscure GI bleeding has been reported to be high [103,104], although the use of double balloon enteroscopy needs to be validated in larger, prospective studies.

Sonde enteroscopy was introduced in 1977 as a method of visualizing the entire small bowel [105–107]. Its role in obscure bleeding has now become extremely limited, in particular given the introduction of double balloon enteroscopy and capsule endoscopy.

Before capsule endoscopy, SBE was generally considered to be the best option for investigation of the small bowel and was considered to be standard in the evaluation of patients with obscure GI bleeding. Its current role is believed to be complementary to that of capsule endoscopy, however, and many experts believe that it should be performed only if capsule endoscopy is positive for a proximal small bowel lesion. The role of double balloon enteroscopy alone or in conjunction with capsule endoscopy requires further study. It is important to emphasize that studies examining the relative roles of each SBE and double balloon enteroscopy in the context of capsule endoscopy have yet to provide an evidence base for the most appropriate test or series of tests. Indeed, the use of these tests likely varies based on individual patient characteristics, and importantly local expertise.

Capsule endoscopy

The GIVEN Diagnostic Imaging System (Given Imaging, Norcross, GA) is currently the only Food and Drug Administration–approved wireless endoscopy system. The Food and Drug Administration approved it in August 2001 as an adjunctive tool for the evaluation of small intestinal diseases and disorders, and subsequently in July 2003, as a first-line modality for evaluation of small bowel disorders. The capsule is swallowed and travels down the GI tract by natural peristalsis. Failure to reach the cecum during the recording period occurs in approximately 20% of patients [108]. The capsule is then naturally excreted in most patients in less than 2 weeks [108]. The first trial comparing capsule endoscopy with push enteroscopy was performed in canines by Appleyard and coworkers [109] in 2000. Radiopaque, colored beads between 3 and 6 mm were sewn into the proximal small bowel of nine dogs. Push enteroscopy and wireless capsule endoscopy, delivered endoscopically into the duodenum, were performed. The sensitivity and specificity of push enteroscopy for detecting beads implanted within the entire small bowel was 37% and 97%, respectively, compared with 64% and 92% for capsule endoscopy. Following this animal study, Appleyard and coworkers [110] reported the first use of capsule endoscopy for obscure GI bleeding in four patients. A diagnosis was made in three patients, two of whom subsequently received endoscopic treatment of vascular lesions. The capsule provided good views and no complications occurred. In an early clinical trial comparing capsule endoscopy and push enteroscopy in patients with obscure GI bleeding [111], 20 patients with obscure GI bleeding underwent both capsule and push enteroscopy. A site of bleeding was found in 55% of patients in the capsule endoscopy group compared with 30% for push enteroscopy ($P = $ NS). Vascular ectasias were the most common finding. Since this time, a number of other studies have examined capsule endoscopy [112–118]. The most common findings were similar, and included vascular lesions, small bowel malignancies, and small bowel ulcerations (Fig. 2). Several studies and dozens of unpublished abstracts have further supported the role of capsule endoscopy in the evaluation of obscure GI bleeding, with an overall diagnostic yield of approximately 55% and 70% [112,115,117,118]. In addition to having a higher yield than SBE, capsule endoscopy also seems to be superior to SBFT and abdominal CT in evaluation of suspected small bowel diseases [113,116]. Capsule endoscopy seems to be most useful for patients with a history of recent active bleeding

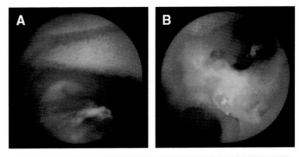

Fig. 2. Examples of lesions found at the time of capsule endoscopy. (A) A patient with recurrent obscure bleeding underwent capsule endoscopy; an ulcer with a red streak over its base, associated with a gastrointestinal stromal tumor in the jejunum, is shown. (B) A patient with recurrent obscure bleeding underwent capsule endoscopy; extensive ulceration was identified in the small bowel. (Courtesy of Brian Dobozi, MD, and Naurang Agrawal, MD, Duke University Medical Center, Durham, NC.)

[108,118,119]. Capsule endoscopy seems to be safe in patients with obscure bleeding. Absolute contraindications for its use include GI obstruction and GI pseudo-obstruction–ileus. Relative contraindications include a history of a GI motility disorder, such as gastroparesis; a history of intestinal strictures or fistula; pregnancy; a known history of multiple small bowel diverticula; a history of Zenker's diverticulum; a history of extensive abdominal surgeries or radiation; an active swallowing disorder or dysphagia; and the presence of a cardiac pacemaker or defibrillator. Although there is concern about the use of capsule endoscopy in patients with pacemakers, evidence suggests capsule endoscopy may be safely performed in these patients [120]. Although the general consensus is that capsule endoscopy has a higher diagnostic yield for small bowel lesions compared with other modalities, it is not completely clear that the findings from capsule endoscopy and subsequent capsule-directed management actually improve patient outcome. Indeed, capsule endoscopy performed in healthy patients finds abnormalities in nearly 23% of cases [121]. This raises an interesting question. Are all abnormalities diagnosed by capsule endoscopy truly significant? In addition, up to 50% of patients suffering from vascular lesions may continue to bleed, even after endoscopic and surgical intervention [98,122]. For capsule endoscopy to be clinically valuable, the higher diagnostic yield should translate into some patient- or physician-perceived benefit, such as reduced transfusion requirements or resolution of bleeding altogether, less need for medical or surgical intervention, reduced medical cost, or improved well-being. For example, several preliminary reports suggest that after capsule endoscopy, clinical improvement reported is limited [123–125]. This area clearly requires further investigation.

Surgery

Exploratory laparotomy is believed to be the last option in the evaluation of obscure GI bleeding. Surgical evaluation can include exploratory laparotomy alone or combined with intraoperative enteroscopy. Studies have shown that laparotomy alone is clearly inferior to the combined approach. In patients with obscure GI bleeding, laparotomy alone leads to a specific diagnosis in 31% to 65% of patients [41,126]. During laparotomy combined with intraoperative enteroscopy, a push enteroscope is used to visualize the small bowel. The surgeon slowly guides the bowel over the endoscope using the air-trapping technique [127]. This is performed by isolating 10 to 15 cm of bowel each time, examining the colon during intubation. If length or extensive air trapping hampers complete visualization of the small bowel from the oral route, retrograde views of the distal ileum by anal intubation should be performed. Unlike standard endoscopy procedures, careful mucosal examination is performed during intubation because trauma (tactile and endoscopic) is induced during endoscope insertion and bowel manipulation. The terminal ileum is reached in more than 90% of patients [128]. Combined with intraoperative enteroscopy, the diagnostic yield has been reported to increase to 50% to 100% [41,122,128–132]. For example, a retrospective study reported a specific diagnosis in 83%

of patients [133,134]. Thirty-four percent had small bowel vascular lesions, followed by 26% with small bowel masses, and 4% with Meckel's diverticulum. Unfortunately, even after surgical intervention, a high proportion of patients rebleed [122,130,131,134]; in a prospective study, a diagnosis was found in 70% of patients [122], leading to partial small bowel resection; unfortunately, 52% of these patients had recurrence of GI bleeding during a mean follow-up of 21 months. Intra-arterial injection of fluorescein during surgery has been suggested to better localize bleeding lesions [135]. It is important to emphasize that exploratory laparotomy is invasive. Serosal tears, postoperative ileus, heart failure, renal failure, and avulsion of superior mesenteric vein have all been reported [128]. Overall, severe complications occur in up to 12% of patients, and mortality can be as high as 8% [134].

TREATMENT

Treatment of patients with obscure bleeding revolves around the etiology of bleeding. Endoscopic, angiographic, and surgical therapy may all be effective. Unfortunately, therapy for the most common finding, vascular ectasias, is often suboptimal and unsatisfactory. Medically treated patients have a rebleeding rate of 26% at 1 year and 46% at 3 years [136]. Patients suffering from a hereditary syndrome, such as Osler-Weber-Rendu, with a high transfusion requirement may have a benefit (lower transfusion requirement) from the administration of estrogen-progesterone [137]. Patients with sporadic lesions seem to have no benefit [138]. Octreotide may lead to decreased transfusion requirements but requires further study [139]. The result of treatment of vascular ectasias with endoscopic therapy has been mixed. Treatment with argon plasma coagulation or electrocautery is highly effective for treatment of acutely bleeding lesions and endoscopic therapy seems to decrease transfusion requirements when compared with no treatment, but rebleeding is common [96,140,141]. Outcomes after surgery are also mixed. One study found that the rebleeding rate was 16% within 1 year and 24% within 3 years compared with 26% and 46%, respectively, for medical management alone [136]. Another study found that surgical treatment was no better than conservative management in decreasing transfusion requirements [136,141]. Importantly, up to 50% of patients receiving endoscopic or surgical therapy may rebleed [94,122,141].

SUMMARY

Obscure GI bleeding is a relatively common problem facing internists, gastroenterologists, and surgeons in a typical clinical practice. The etiology is occasionally suggested by the patient's age, history, and medications. Management is complicated and typically requires a team-oriented approach, with input from the internist, gastroenterologist, radiologist, and surgeon alike. SBFT and enteroclysis seem to have a limited role, unless there is a high suspicion of a small bowel mass lesion or Crohn's disease. Scintigraphy may be performed in patients with active bleeding in whom endoscopy has failed or is contraindicated. Angiography may be used in patients with an early positive nuclear imaging or failed endoscopic therapy. Provocative angiography probably has a lower diagnostic yield than previously reported, and should be performed only in experienced centers. Helical CT is a new and potentially important option in patients with obscure bleeding, but is currently considered experimental. All patients with obscure GI bleeding should undergo repeat upper endoscopy and perhaps colonoscopy to rule out missed lesions. SBE seems to be complementary to capsule endoscopy, and it is unknown whether this should be performed before capsule endoscopy or only if capsule endoscopy yields a positive proximal small bowel finding. Double balloon enteroscopy seems promising, but the technique requires further study. Surgery should be reserved for patients who have a positive capsule endoscopy requiring surgical therapy or patients who have persistent GI bleeding requiring recurrent blood transfusions in whom all other modalities have failed. Treatment for vascular ectasias, the most common cause of obscure GI bleeding, is currently inadequate, and typically requires a combination of multiple management approaches.

References

[1] AGA. American gastroenterological association medical position statement: evaluation and management of occult and obscure gastrointestinal bleeding. Gastroenterology 2000;118:197.

[2] Spiller RC, Parkins RA. Recurrent gastrointestinal bleeding of obscure origin: report of 17 cases and a guide to logical management. Br J Surg 1983;70:489.

[3] Thompson JN, Salem RR, Hemingway AP, et al. Specialist investigation of obscure gastrointestinal bleeding. Gut 1987;28:47.

[4] ASGE. Obscure gastrointestinal bleeding. Gastrointest Endosc 2003;58:650.

[5] Lewis BS. Small intestinal bleeding. Gastroenterol Clin North Am 1994;23:67.

[6] Mujica VR, Barkin JS. Occult gastrointestinal bleeding: general overview and approach. Gastrointest Endosc Clin N Am 1996;6:833.

[7] Hilsman JH. The color of blood-containing feces following the instillation of citrated blood at various levels of the small intestine. Gastroenterology 1950;15:131.

[8] Chak A, Koehler MK, Sundaram SN, et al. Diagnostic and therapeutic impact of push enteroscopy: analysis of factors associated with positive findings. Gastrointest Endosc 1998;47:18.

[9] O'Mahony S, Morris AJ, Straiton M, et al. Push enteroscopy in the investigation of small-intestinal disease. QJM 1996;89:685.

[10] Zaman A, Katon RM. Push enteroscopy for obscure gastrointestinal bleeding yields a high incidence of proximal lesions within reach of a standard endoscope. Gastrointest Endosc 1998;47:372.

[11] Waye JD. Enteroscopy. Gastrointest Endosc 1997;46:247.

[12] Rollins ES, Picus D, Hicks ME, et al. Angiography is useful in detecting the source of chronic gastrointestinal bleeding of obscure origin. AJR Am J Roentgenol 1991;156:385.

[13] Lewis BS, Kornbluth A, Waye JD. Small bowel tumours: yield of enteroscopy. Gut 1991;32:763.

[14] Maglinte DDT, Kelvin FM, O'Connor K, et al. Current status of small bowel radiography. Abdom Imaging 1996;21:247.

[15] Rabe FE, Becker GJ, Besozzi MJ, et al. Efficacy study of the small-bowel examination. Radiology 1981;140:47.

[16] Fried AM, Poulos A, Hatfield DR. The effectiveness of the incidental small-bowel series. Radiology 1981;140:45.

[17] Foutch PG, Sawyer R, Sanowski RA. Push-enteroscopy for diagnosis of patients with gastrointestinal bleeding of obscure origin. Gastrointest Endosc 1990;36:337.

[18] Lewis BS, Waye JD. Undiagnosed chronic occult GI bleeding: the role of total small-bowel enteroscopy. A new diagnostic tool. Am J Gastroenterol 1986;81:AB858.

[19] Kusumoto H, Takahashi I, Yoshida M, et al. Primary malignant tumors of the small intestine: analysis of 40 Japanese patients. J Surg Oncol 1992;50:139.

[20] Bernstein CN, Boult IF, Greenberg HM, et al. A prospective randomized comparison between small bowel enteroclysis and small bowel follow-through in Crohn's disease. Gastroenterology 1997;113:390.

[21] Carlson HC. Perspective: the small-bowel examination in the diagnosis of Crohn's disease. AJR Am J Roentgenol 1986;147:63.

[22] Ott DJ, Chen YM, Gerlfand DW, et al. Detailed per-oral small bowel examination vs. enteroclysis. Radiology 1985;155:29.

[23] Maglinte DDT, Elmore MF, Chernish SM, et al. Enteroclysis in the diagnosis of chronic unexplained gastrointestinal bleeding. Dis Colon Rectum 1985;28:403.

[24] Moch A, Herlinger H, Kochman ML, et al. Enteroclysis in the evaluation of obscure gastrointestinal bleeding. AJR Am J Roentgenol 1994;163:1381.

[25] Rex DK, Lappas JC, Maglinte DDT, et al. Enteroclysis in the evaluation of suspected small intestinal bleeding. Gastroenterology 1989;97:58.

[26] Bessette JR, Maglinte DDT, Kelvin FM, et al. Primary malignant tumors in the small bowel: a comparison of the small-bowel enema and conventional follow-through examination. AJR Am J Roentgenol 1989;153:741.

[27] Maglinte DD, Chernish SM, Kelvin FM, et al. Crohn disease of the small intestine: accuracy and relevance of enteroclysis. Radiology 1992;184:541.

[28] Chernish SM, Maglinte DD, O'Connor K. Evaluation of the small intestine by enteroclysis for Crohn's disease. Am J Gastroenterol 1992;87:696.

[29] Vallance R. An evaluation of the small bowel enema based on an analysis of 350 consecutive examinations. Clin Radiol 1980;31:227.

[30] Bernstein CN. A prospective randomized comparison between small bowel enteroclysis and small bowel follow-through in Crohn's disease [letter reply]. Gastroenterology 1998;114:1350.

[31] Gasche C, Schober E, Turetschek K. Small bowel barium studies in Crohn's disease. Gastroenterology 1998;114:1349.

[32] Kelvin FM, Maglinte DD. Enteroclysis or small bowel follow-through in Crohn's disease? Gastroenterology 1998;114:1349–51.

[33] Nolan DJ. Small bowel enteroclysis: pros. Abdom Imaging 1996;21:243.

[34] Howarth DM, Tang K, Lees W. The clinical utility of nuclear medicine imaging for the detection of occult gastrointestinal haemorrhage. Nucl Med (Stuttg) 2002;23:591.

[35] McKusick KA, Froelich J, Callahan RJ, et al. 99mTc red blood cells for detection of gastrointestinal bleeding: experience with 80 patients. AJR Am J Roentgenol 1981;137: 1113.

[36] Ohri SK, Desa LA, Lee H, et al. Value of scintigraphic localization of obscure gastrointestinal bleeding. J R Coll Surg Edinb 1992;37:328.

[37] Szasz IJ, Morrison RT, Lyster DM. Technetium-99m-labelled red blood cell scanning to diagnose occult gastrointestinal bleeding. Can J Surg 1985;28:512.

[38] Voeller GR, Bunch G, Britt LG. Use of technetium-labeled red blood cell scintigraphy in the detection and management of gastrointestinal hemorrhage. Surgery 1991;110:799.

[39] Wang CS, Tzen KY, Huang MJ, et al. Localization of obscure gastrointestinal bleeding by technetium 99m-labeled red blood cell scintigraphy. J Formos Med Assoc 1992;91:63.

[40] Hunter JM, Pezim ME. Limited value of the technetium-99m-labeled red cell scintigraphy in localization of lower gastrointestinal bleeding. Am J Surg 1990;159:504.

[41] Wells SA. Occult and obscure sources of gastrointestinal bleeding. Curr Probl Surg 2000;37:863.

[42] Ng DA, Opelka FG, Beck DE, et al. Predictive value of technetium Tc 99m-labeled red blood cell scintigraphy for positive angiogram in massive lower gastrointestinal hemorrhage. Dis Colon Rectum 1997;40:471.

[43] Ymaguchi M, Takeuchi S, Awazu S. Meckel's diverticulum: investigation of 600 patients in Japanese literature. Am J Surg 1978;136:247.

[44] Berman EJ, Schneider A, Potts WJ. Importance of gastric mucosa in Meckel's diverticulum. JAMA 1954;156:6.

[45] Schwartz MJ, Lewis JH. Meckel's diverticulum: pitfalls in scintigraphic detection in the adult. Am J Gastroenterol 1984;79:611.

[46] Kong MS, Chen CY, Tzen KY, et al. Technetium-99m pertechnetate scan for ectopic gastric mucosa in children with gastrointestinal bleeding. J Formos Med Assoc 1993;92:717.

[47] Sfakianakis GN, Conway JJ. Detection of ectopic gastric mucosa in Meckel's diverticulum and in other aberrations by scintigraphy: II. Indications and methods- a 10-year experience. J Nucl Med 1981;22:732.

[48] Kong MS, Huang SC, Tzen KY, et al. Repeated technetium-99m pertechnetate scanning for children with obscure gastrointestinal bleeding. J Pediatr Gastr Nutr 1994;18:284.

[49] Lin S, Suhocki PV, Ludwig KA, et al. Gastrointestinal bleeding in adult patients with Meckel's diverticulum: the role of technetium 99m pertechnetate scan. South Med J 2002;95:1338.

[50] Heyman S. Meckel's diverticulum: possible detection by combining pentagastrin with histamine H2 receptor blocker. J Nucl Med 1994;35:1656.

[51] Treves S, Grand RJ, Eraklis AJ. Pentagastrin stimulation of technetium-99m uptake by ectopic gastric mucosa in a Meckel's diverticulum. Radiology 1978;128:711.

[52] Diamond RH, Rothstein RD, Alavi A. The role of cimetidine-enhanced technetium-99m-pertechnetate imaging for visualizing Meckel's diverticulum. J Nucl Med 1991;32:1422.

[53] Petrakubi RJ, Baum S, Rahrer GV. Cimetidine administration resulting in improved pertechnetate imaging of Meckel's diverticulum. Clin Nucl Med 1978;3:385.

[54] Singh PR, Russell CD, Dubovsky EV, et al. Technique of scanning for Meckel's diverticulum. Clin Nucl Med 1978;3:188.

[55] Connolly LP, Treves ST, Bozorgi F, et al. Meckel's diverticulum: demonstration of heterotopic gastric mucosa with technetium-99m-pertechnetate SPECT. J Nucl Med 1998;39:1458.

[56] Lau WY, Fan ST, Wong SH, et al. Preoperative and intraoperative localisation of gastrointestinal bleeding of obscure origin. Gut 1987;28:869.

[57] Nusbaum M, Baum S, Blakemore WS. Clinical experience with the diagnosis and management of gastrointestinal haemorrhage by selective mesenteric catheterization. Ann Surg 1969;170:506.

[58] Moore JD, Thompson NW, Appleman HD, et al. Arteriovenous malformations of the gastrointestinal tract. Arch Surg 1976;111:381.

[59] Lau WY, Ngan H, Chu KW, et al. Repeat selective visceral angiography in patients with gastrointestinal bleeding of obscure origin. Br J Surg 1989;76:226.

[60] Sheedy FP, Fulton RE, Atwell DT. Angiographic evaluation of patients with chronic gastrointestinal bleeding. AJR Am J Roentgenol 1975;123:338.

[61] Ng BL, Thompson JN, Adam A, et al. Selective visceral angiography in obscure postoperative gastrointestinal bleeding. Ann R Coll Surg Engl 1987;69:237.

[62] Cohn SM, Moller BA, Zieg PM, et al. Angiography for preoperative evaluation in patients with lower gastrointestinal bleeding: are the benefits worth the risks? Arch Surg 1998;133:50.

[63] Baum S, Rosch J, Dotter CT, et al. Selective mesenteric arterial infusions in the management of massive diverticular hemorrhage. N Engl J Med 1973;288:1269.

[64] Browder W, Cerise EJ, Litwin MS. Impact of emergency angiography in massive lower gastrointestinal bleeding. Ann Surg 1986;204:530.

[65] Eckstein MR, Kelemouridis V, Athanasoulis CA, et al. Gastric bleeding: therapy with intraarterial vasopressin and transcatheter embolization. Radiology 1984;152:643.

[66] Funaki B. Endovascular intervention for the treatment of acute arterial gastrointestinal bleeding. Gastroenterol Clin North Am 2002;31:701.

[67] Bloomfield RS, Smith TP, Schneider AM, et al. Provocative angiography in patients with gastrointestinal hemorrhage of obscure origin. Am J Gastroenterol 2000;95:2807.

[68] Koval G, Benner KG, Rosch J, et al. Aggressive angiographic diagnosis in acute lower gastrointestinal hemorrhage. Dig Dis Sci 1987;32:248.

[69] Malden ES, Hicks ME, Royal HD, et al. Recurrent gastrointestinal bleeding: use of thrombolysis with anticoagulation in diagnosis. Radiology 1998;207:147.

[70] Mernagh JR, O'Donovan N, Somers S, et al. Use of heparin in the investigation of obscure gastrointestinal bleeding. Gastrointest Radiol 2001;52:232.

[71] Rosch J, Kozak BE, Keller FS, et al. Interventional angiography in the diagnosis of acute lower gastrointestinal bleeding. Eur J Radiol 1986;6:136.

[72] Ettorre GC, Francioso G, Garribba AP, et al. Helical CT angiography in gastrointestinal bleeding of obscure origin. AJR Am J Roentgenol 1997;168:727.

[73] Junquera F, Quiroga S, Saperas E, et al. Accuracy of helical computed tomographic angiography for the diagnosis of colonic angiodysplasia. Gastroenterology 2000; 119:293.

[74] Kuhle WG, Engr MS, Sheiman RG. Detection of active colonic hemorrhage with use of helical CT: findings in a swine model. Radiology 2003;228:743.

[75] Summers RM. Science to practice: detection of active colonic hemorrhage with use of helical CT: findings in a swine model. Radiology 2003;228:599.

[76] Miller FH, Hwang CM. An initial experience: using helical CT imaging to detect obscure gastrointestinal bleeding. Clin Imaging 2004;28:245.

[77] Miller FH, Kline MJ, Vanagunas AD. Detection of bleeding due to small bowel cholesterol emboli using helical CT examination in gastrointestinal bleeding of obscure origin. Am J Gastroenterol 1999;94:3623.

[78] Ernst O, Bulois P, Saint-Drenant S, et al. Helical CT in acute lower gastrointestinal bleeding. Eur Radiol 2003;13:114.

[79] Kim KW, Ha HK. MRI for small bowel diseases. Semin Ultrasound CT 2003;24:387.

[80] Descamps C, Schmit A, Van Gossum A. "Missed" upper gastrointestinal tract lesions may explain "occult" bleeding. Endoscopy 1999;31:452.

[81] Lin S, Branch MS, Shetzline M. The importance of indication in the diagnostic value of push enteroscopy. Endoscopy 2003;35:315.

[82] Ackerman Z, Eliakim R, Stalnikowicz R, et al. Role of small bowel biopsy in the endoscopic evaluation of adults with iron deficiency anemia. Am J Gastroenterol 1996;91:2099.

[83] Carroccio A, Iannitto E, Cavataio F, et al. Sideropenic anemia and celiac disease: one study, two points of view. Dig Dis Sci 1998;43:673.

[84] Lewis BS. The history of enteroscopy. Gastrointest Endosc Clin N Am 1999;9:1.

[85] Ogoshi K, Hara Y, Ashizawa S. New technic for small intestinal fiberoscopy. Gastrointest Endosc 1973;20:64.

[86] Parker HW, Agayoff JD. Enteroscopy and small bowel biopsy utilizing a peroral colonoscope [letter]. Gastrointest Endosc 1983;29:139.

[87] Benz C, Jakobs R, Riemann JF. Do we need overtube for push enteroscopy? Endoscopy 2001;33:658.

[88] Cotton P, Williams C. Practical gastrointestinal endoscopy. 4th edition. Oxford: Blackwell Science; 1996.

[89] Taylor AC, Chen RY, Desmond PV. Use of an overtube for enteroscopy: does it increase depth of insertion? A prospective study of enteroscopy with and without overtube. Endoscopy 2001;33:227.

[90] Wilmer A, Rutgeerts P. Push enteroscopy: technique, depth, and yield of insertion. Gastrointest Endosc Clin N Am 1996;6:759.

[91] Yang R, Laine L. Mucosal stripping: a complication of push enteroscopy. Gastrointest Endosc 1995;41:156.

[92] Adrain AL, Dabezies MA, Krevsky B. Enteroscopy improves the clinical outcome in patients with obscure gastrointestinal bleeding. J Laparoendosc Adv Surg Tech A 1998;8:279.

[93] Chong J, Tagle M, Barkin JS, et al. Small bowel push-type fiberoptic enteroscopy for patients with occult gastrointestinal bleeding or suspected small bowel pathology. Am J Gastroenterol 1994;89:2143.

[94] Landi B, Tkoub M, Gaudric M, et al. Diagnostic yield of push-type enteroscopy in relation to indication. Gut 1998;42:421.

[95] Rossini FP, Arrigoni A, Pennazio M. Clinical enteroscopy. J Clin Gastroenterol 1996;22:231.

[96] Schmit A, Gay F, Adler M, et al. Diagnostic efficacy of push-enteroscopy and long-term follow-up of patients with small bowel angiodysplasias. Dig Dis Sci 1996;41:2348.

[97] Sharma BC, Bhasin DK, Makharia G, et al. Diagnostic value of push-type enteroscopy: a report from India. Am J Gastroenterol 2000;95:137.

[98] Landi B, Cellier C, Gaudric M, et al. Long-term outcome of patients with gastrointestinal bleeding of obscure origin explored by push enteroscopy. Endoscopy 2002;34:355.

[99] Shinozaki S, Yamamoto H, Kita H, et al. Direct observation with double-balloon enteroscopy of an intestinal intramural hematoma resulting in anticoagulant ileus. Dig Dis Sci 2004;49:902.

[100] Yamamoto H, Sekine Y, Sato Y, et al. Total enteroscopy with a nonsurgical steerable double-balloon method. Gastrointest Endosc 2001;53:216.

[101] Yamamoto H, Sugano K. A new method of enteroscopy-the double-balloon method. Can J Gastroenterol 2003;17:273.

[102] Yamamoto H, Yano T, Kita H, et al. New system of double-balloon enteroscopy for diagnosis and treatment of small intestinal disorders. Gastroenterology 1556;2003:125.

[103] May A, Nachbar L, Wardak A, et al. Double-balloon enteroscopy: preliminary experience in patients with obscure gastrointestinal bleeding or chronic abdominal pain. Endoscopy 2003;35:985.

[104] Yamamoto H, Kita H, Sunada K, et al. Clinical outcomes of double-balloon endoscopy for the diagnosis and treatment of small-intestinal diseases. Clin Gastroenterol Hepatol 2004;2:1010.

[105] Berner JS, Mauer K, Lewis BS. Push and sonde enteroscopy for the diagnosis of obscure gastrointestinal bleeding. Am J Gastroenterol 1994;89:2139.

[106] Lewis BS, Waye JD. Chronic gastrointestinal bleeding of obscure origin: role of small bowel enteroscopy. Gastroenterology 1988;94:1117.

[107] Seensalu R. The sonde examination. Gastrointest Endosc Clin N Am 1999;9:37.

[108] Pennazio M, Santucci R, Rondonotti E, et al. Outcome of patients with obscure gastrointestinal bleeding after capsule endoscopy: report of 100 consecutive cases. Gastroenterology 2004;126:643.

[109] Appleyard M, Zireman Z, Glukhovsky A, et al. A randomized trial comparing wireless capsule endoscopy with push enteroscopy for detection of small-bowel lesions. Gastroenterology 2000;119:1431.

[110] Appleyard M, Glukhovsky A, Swain P. Wireless-capsule diagnostic endoscopy for recurrent small-bowel bleeding. N Engl J Med 2001;344:232.

[111] Lewis B, Swain P. Capsule endoscopy in the evaluation of patients with suspected small intestinal bleeding: results of a pilot study. Gastrointest Endosc 2002;56:349.

[112] Chong AK, Taylor AC, Miller AM, et al. Initial experience of capsule endoscopy at a major referral center. Med J Aust 2003;178:537.

[113] Costamagna G, Shah SK, Riccioni ME, et al. A prospective trial comparing small bowel radiographs and video capsule endoscopy for suspected small bowel disease. Gastroenterology 2002;123:999.

[114] Ell C, Remke S, May A, et al. The first prospective controlled trial comparing wireless capsule endoscopy with push enteroscopy in chronic gastrointestinal bleeding. Endoscopy 2002;34:685.

[115] Hahne M, Adamek HE, Schilling D, et al. Wireless capsule endoscopy in a patient with obscure occult bleeding. Endoscopy 2002;34:588.

[116] Hara AK, Leighton JA, Sharma VK, et al. Small bowel: preliminary comparison of capsule endoscopy with barium study and CT. Radiology 2004;230:260.

[117] Mylonaki M, Fritscher-Ravens A, Swain P. Wireless capsule endoscopy: a comparison with push enteroscopy in patients with gastroscopy and colonoscopy negative gastrointestinal bleeding. Gut 2003;52:1122.

[118] Saurin JC, Delvaux M, Gaudin JL, et al. Diagnostic value of endoscopic capsule in patients with obscure digestive bleeding: blinded comparison with video push-enteroscopy. Endoscopy 2003;35:576.

[119] Selby W. Can clinical features predict the likelihood of finding abnormalities when using capsule endoscopy in patients with GI bleeding of obscure origin? Gastrointest Endosc 2004;59:782.

[120] Leighton JA, Sharma VK, Srivathsan K, et al. Safety of capsule endoscopy in patients with pacemakers. Gastrointest Endosc 2004;59:567.

[121] Goldstein J, Eisen G, Lewis B, et al. Abnormal small bowel findings are common in healthy subjects screened for a multi-center, double blind, randomized, placebo-controlled trial using capsule endoscopy. Gastroenterology 2003;124:A37.

[122] Ress AM, Bennacci JC, Sarr MG. Efficacy of intraoperative enteroscopy in diagnosis and prevention of recurrent, occult gastrointestinal bleeding. Am J Surg 1992;163:94.

[123] Chong A, Taylor A, Miller A, et al. Clinical outcomes following capsule endoscopy (CE) examination of patients with obscure gastrointestinal bleeding (OGB). Gastrointest Endosc 2003;57:AB166.

[124] Chutkan R, Toubia N, Balba N. Findings and follow-up on the first 125 video capsule patients at Georgetown University Hospital. Gastrointest Endosc 2003;57:AB85.

[125] Rostogi A, Schoen RE, Silivka A. Diagnostic yield and outcomes of capsule endoscopy. Gastrointest Endosc 2003;57:AB163.

[126] Brearley S, Hawker PC, Dorricott NJ, et al. The importance of laparotomy in the diagnosis and management of intestinal bleeding of obscure origin. Ann R Coll Surg Engl 1986;68:245.

[127] Delmotte JS, Gay GJ, Houcke PH, et al. Intraoperative endoscopy. Gastrointest Endosc Clin N Am 1999;9:61.

[128] Zaman A, Sheppard B, Katon RM. Total peroral intraoperative enteroscopy for obscure GI bleeding using a dedicated push enteroscope: diagnostic yield and patient outcome. Gastrointest Endosc 1999;50:506.

[129] Desa LA, Ohri SK, Hutton KA, et al. Role of intraoperative enteroscopy in obscure gastrointestinal bleeding of small bowel origin. Br J Surg 1991;78:192.

[130] Douard R, Wind P, Panis Y, et al. Intraoperative enteroscopy for diagnosis and management of unexplained gastrointestinal bleeding. Am J Surg 2000;180:181.

[131] Lewis BS, Wenger JS, Waye JD. Small bowel enteroscopy and intraoperative enteroscopy for obscure gastrointestinal bleeding. Am J Gastroenterol 1991;86:171.

[132] Szold A, Katz LB, Lewis BS. Surgical approach to occult gastrointestinal bleeding. Am J Surg 1992;163:90.

[133] Baillie JB. Value of laparotomy in the diagnosis of obscure gastrointestinal haemorrhage. Gastrointest Endosc 1997;45:219.

[134] Lewis MPN, Khoo DE, Spencer J. Value of laparotomy in the diagnosis of obscure gastrointestinal haemorrhage. Gut 1995;37:187.

[135] Ohri SK, Jackson J, Desa LA, et al. The intraoperative localization of the obscure bleeding site using fluorescein. J Clin Gastroenterol 1992;14:331.

[136] Richter JM, Christensen MR, Colditz GA, et al. Angiodysplasia: natural history and efficacy of therapeutic interventions. Dig Dis Sci 1989;34:1542.

[137] van Cutsem E, Rutgeerts P, Vantrappen G. Treatment of bleeding gastrointestinal vascular malformations with oestrogen-progesterone. Lancet 1990;335:953.

[138] Junquera F, Feu F, Papo M, et al. A multicenter, randomized, clinical trial of hormonal therapy in the prevention of rebleeding from gastrointestinal angiodysplasia. Gastroenterology
2002;121:1073.
[139] Nardone G, Rocco A, Balzano T, et al. The efficacy of octreotide therapy in chronic bleeding due to vascular abnormalities of the gastrointestinal tract. Aliment Pharmacol Ther
1999;13:1429.
[140] Askin MP, Lewis BS. Push enteroscopic cauterization: long-term follow-up of 83 patients
with bleeding small intestinal andiodysplasia. Gastrointest Endosc 1996;43:580.
[141] Hutcheon DF, Kabelin J, Bulkley GB, et al. Effect of therapy on bleeding rates in gastrointestinal angiodysplasia. Am Surg 1987;53:6.

Gastroenterol Clin N Am 34 (2005) 699–718

GASTROENTEROLOGY CLINICS
OF NORTH AMERICA

Occult Gastrointestinal Bleeding

Don C. Rockey, MD

Division of Digestive and Liver Diseases, University of Texas Southwestern Medical Center,
5323 Harry Hines Boulevard, Dallas, TX 75390, USA

The potential frequency of unrecognized or occult gastrointestinal bleeding is emphasized by the observation that instillation of 150 to 200 mL into the stomach is required to consistently produce visible evidence of blood in the stool (ie, melena) [1]. Additionally, patients with gastroduodenal bleeding of up to 100 mL per day may have normal-appearing stools. Thus, occult bleeding often is identified only by fecal occult blood tests that detect fecal blood, or, if bleeding occurs for a long enough period of time, it may become manifest as by iron depletion and anemia.

IRON DEFICIENCY ANEMIA

Iron deficiency is the most common cause of anemia in the world, and it is most prevalent in neonates and in young children. Although iron deficiency is less prevalent in adults than in children, it remains extremely common. In the United States alone, 5% to 11% of women and 1% to 4% of men are iron deficient; approximately 5% and 2% of adult women and men, respectively, have iron deficiency anemia [2]. Iron deficiency anemia is most common in women during their reproductive years because of menstrual and pregnancy-associated iron losses [3]. In groups other than premenopausal women, iron deficiency anemia traditionally has been assumed to be caused by chronic occult gastrointestinal bleeding. Thus, the standard of care for men and postmenopausal women with iron deficiency anemia is to investigate the gastrointestinal tract [4].

Iron Metabolism

Iron balance is regulated tightly under normal physiologic conditions (Fig. 1). The primary means that the body maintains iron balance is by regulation of iron absorption, a process that appears to be extremely complex [5]. The reliable absorptive process allows an increase in absorption of iron by several-fold in response to iron depletion. Obligate daily fecal blood loss (under normal

E-mail address: don.rockey@utsouthwestern.edu

0889-8553/05/$ – see front matter
doi:10.1016/j.gtc.2005.08.010

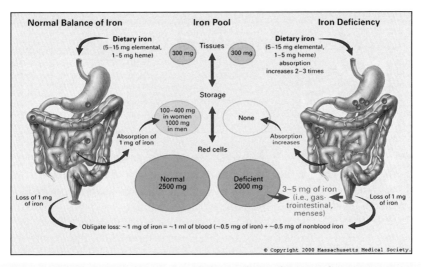

Fig. 1. Gastrointestinal blood loss and iron balance. The usual Western diet contains 5 to 15 mg of elemental iron and 1 to 5 mg of heme-iron, of which about 10% are absorbed. Heme-iron, derived primary from myoglobin in meats, is absorbed preferentially and accounts for 60% to 80% of the iron absorbed per day. Iron loss of approximately 0.5 mg (1 mL of blood assuming a normal hemoglobin) per day results from occult bleeding in the form of microerosions or microulcerations in the gastrointestinal tract. Additionally, small amounts of iron are lost from sloughing of gut epithelial cells (with iron-containing proteins). Altogether, iron loss is approximately 1 mg/d. Under normal circumstances, iron homeostasis is regulated tightly, and daily iron loss is balanced precisely by small bowel iron absorption. Normal iron balance can be maintained even in the face of small additional amounts of iron loss. In pathologic states, however, even though the absorptive capacity of the small bowel increases two- to threefold during states of iron depletion, if blood loss exceeds the compensatory capacity of the small bowel, depletion of total body iron stores ensues, ultimately leading to iron deficiency anemia. The time required to develop iron deficiency depends on the size of initial iron stores, intestinal iron absorption and the rate of bleeding. Iron deficiency anemia occurs only after storage iron is exhausted and is thus a late manifestation of the iron depleted state. Additionally, iron absorption and homeostasis may be confounded by the amount of iron in the diet or intrinsic disease of the gastrointestinal tract, such as atrophic gastritis, which may impair iron absorption and may even contribute to primary iron imbalance. (*From* Rockey DC. Occult gastrointestinal bleeding. N Engl J Med 1999;341:38–46. © 1999 Massachusetts Medical Society. All rights reserved; with permission.)

conditions) varies from 0.5 to 1.5 mL per day [6,7]. Therefore, given a typical daily stool weight of 150 g and a circulating hemoglobin level of 15 g/dL, the usual stool hemoglobin concentration is thus 0.5 to 1.5 mg per gram stool, corresponding to a total of 0.25 to 0.75 mg of elemental iron. In addition, a small amount of iron is lost by means sloughing of intestinal epithelial cells, a highly dynamic process. All told, usual iron loss is approximately 1 mg/d (see Fig. 1). Iron deficiency results when the absorptive capacity of the small intestine (which increases to a maximum of two- to fourfold above normal) is exceeded by iron loss over a prolonged period of time.

Differential Diagnosis

The diagnosis of iron deficiency and iron deficiency anemia should be considered any time that a low serum hemoglobin level or hematocrit is encountered. A reduced mean corpuscular volume (MCV) supports the diagnosis, but is not definitive. Caution is required when considering the diagnosis of iron deficiency anemia with only a low hemoglobin or MCV in hand, because numerous diseases can lead to microcytosis. Caution also is required when using iron and transferrin saturation to make a definitive diagnosis of iron deficiency anemia, especially in the setting of a low serum transferrin (ie, below 200 mg/dL). The diagnosis is confirmed most readily by documenting a low serum ferritin level. Serum ferritin is an excellent test with which to investigate iron deficiency anemia; it is relatively sensitive and specific for the diagnosis [8] and should be the first test ordered when investigating presumed iron deficiency anemia. A very low ferritin level (less than 20 ng/mL) is essentially diagnostic of iron deficiency anemia. Notably, when ferritin levels are between 20 and 45 ng/mL, iron deficiency anemia is likely. Additionally, with serum ferritin levels between 45 and 100 ng/mL, iron deficiency anemia still can exist, especially in situations where inflammation is present. When diagnosis of iron deficiency is uncertain, bone marrow examination should be considered. Because a diagnosis of iron deficiency anemia in postmenopausal women or men will lead to extensive and often costly evaluation, it is important that the diagnosis of iron deficiency anemia be established carefully.

Approach to Evaluation

Essentially any lesion in the gastrointestinal tract can bleed in an occult fashion and lead to iron deficiency anemia (Table 1). Historically, iron deficiency anemia has been thought to be associated with right-sided colon cancer (because cancers in the right colon may not become symptomatic, and their bleeding can remain undetected for long periods of time). Many studies, however, have documented a high frequency of abnormalities in the upper gastrointestinal tract [9–18]. Data from four of the larger series are shown in Table 2 and emphasize the point that upper gastrointestinal lesions such as severe esophagitis (presumably reflux-mediated), gastric or duodenal ulcer, and gastric cancer can be identified commonly in patients with iron deficiency anemia. Additionally, small intestinal abnormalities may be present in patients with iron deficiency anemia. Identification of synchronous lesions potentially responsible for iron deficiency anemia is uncommon.

Studies such as those highlighted in Table 2 have helped change the way patients with iron deficiency anemia are managed, in particular, emphasizing evaluation of the upper gastrointestinal tract and small bowel. A critical issue in managing patients with iron deficiency anemia, however, is that the clinician must correlate gastrointestinal lesions with the degree of blood loss appropriately. For example, although it is clear that mass lesions and large ulcerative upper gastrointestinal lesions can lead to substantial blood loss (up to 20 mL/d) [6,19] of the magnitude required to lead to iron deficiency anemia, it

Table 1
Differential diagnosis of occult gastrointestinal bleeding (iron deficiency anemia or fecal occult blood)

Mass lesions	Vascular
[1]Carcinoma (any site)	[1]Vascular ectasia (any site)
Large (>1.5 cm) adenoma (any site)	Portal hypertensive gastropathy/colopathy
Inflammation	Watermelon stomach
[1]Erosive esophagitis	Hemangioma
[1]Ulcer (any site)	[3]Dieulafoy's ulcer
[2]Cameron lesions	Infectious
Erosive gastritis	Hookworm
Celiac sprue	Whipworm
Ulcerative colitis	Stronglyoidiasis
Crohn's disease	Ascariasis
Colitis (nonspecific)	Tuberculous enterocolitis
Idiopathic cecal ulcer	Amebiasis
Miscellaneous	Surreptitious
Long-distance running	Hemoptysis
Factitious	Oropharyngeal (including epistaxis)
Pancreaticobiliary	

Some lesions that may lead to recurrent obscure bleeding are not listed.
  Potential lesions leading to all forms of occult gastrointestinal bleeding are shown.
  [1]Most common abnormalities.
  [2]Linear erosions within a hiatus hernia.
  [3]Large superficial artery underlying mucosal defect.
  Adapted from Rockey DC. Occult gastrointestinal bleeding. N Engl J Med 1999;341:38–46. © 1999 Massachusetts Medical Society. All rights reserved; with permission.

is unlikely that trivial lesions (such as mild inflammation and especially small adenomas) bleed enough to lead to iron deficiency. Thus, judgment must be used when linking certain gastrointestinal tract lesions to iron deficiency anemia. This point is emphasized by a study that demonstrated that although two-thirds of patients with iron deficiency anemia had identifiable gastrointestinal tract lesions, elevated hemoglobin levels in gastrointestinal lavage specimens were detected in only 19% of patients [20]. Although this study is confounded by daily variability in gastrointestinal bleeding (and one-time gastrointestinal blood measurements were performed in this study), the point that every lesion identified in the gastrointestinal tract is not necessarily associated with occult bleeding and iron deficiency is emphasized.

Some patients who have iron deficiency anemia will have gastrointestinal symptoms, while others may not [4,18,21]. In those who have symptoms, these symptoms may help focus evaluation to one specific area of the gastrointestinal tract [13,17,22]. Others, however, have found that symptoms are not helpful in localizing pathology [14,16]. Focusing gastrointestinal tract evaluation has obvious benefits. Classic symptoms such as change in stool caliber or epigastric pain should focus the evaluation initially. Subtle symptoms also should be elicited (ie, weight loss, early satiety, poor appetite, or change in bowel habit). It is this author's belief that the initial investigation should be directed toward the

Table 2
Major gastrointestinal lesions identified in studies of patients with iron deficiency anemia

| | Author (total # of patients evaluable) | | | | |
Lesion	[1]Cook (100)	[1]McIntyre (111)	Rockey (100)	Kepczyk (70)	Total (381)
Esophagus (%)					47
Esophagitis	14	15	6	10	
Cancer	1	na	0	1	
Stomach					98
Ulcer	7	13	8	3	
Gastritis	[2]14	7	6	11	
Cancer	5	8	1	3	
Vascular ectasia	5	0	3	4	
Duodenal ulcer	1	10	11	3	25
Other upper small intestine	0	2	2	3	7
					10
[3]Celiac dis.	0	3	0	4	
Vascular ectasia	1	1	0	0	
Large intestine					85
Cancer	14	5	11	4	
Vascular ectasia	2	1	5	6	
Adenoma	6	4	5	6	
Colitis	1	2	2	1	
Other	0	3	3	4	
[4]Upper lesion	40 (47)	42 (51)	37	39 (43)	158 (41%)
Lower lesion	23	15	26	21	85 (22%)
Small intestine	2	4	0	4	10 (3%)
Upper and lower	7	0	1	12	20 (5%)
No gastrointestinal lesion	35	50	37	6	128 (34%)

Numbers shown are the reported lesions. Hiatal hernia alone, esophageal varices alone, and hemorrhoids alone were not included as sources of chronic blood loss.

[1]Barium enema was used to evaluate the colon in many patients.

[2]Duodenitis included.

[3]Duodenal biopsy was not performed to evaluate for celiac disease in all patients.

[4]Numbers shown represent those patients with abnormalities identified. The numbers in parentheses represent the number of reported lesions. For example, 47 lesions were identified in 40 patients by Cook and colleagues.

Data from Rockey DC. Gastrointestinal bleeding. In: Feldman M, Friedman LS, Sleisenger MH, editors. Sleisenger & Fordtran's gastrointestinal and liver disease. 7th edition. Philadelphia: Saunders; 2002. p. 211–48.

location of specific symptoms, either upper or lower gastrointestinal tract (Fig. 2). Because synchronous lesions are rare, identification of an obvious abnormality clearly associated with chronic bleeding (ie, such as a mass lesion, large ulceration, or severe inflammation) makes further evaluation unnecessary. In the absence of symptoms, particularly in elderly patients, evaluation should begin with the colon, but if this is negative, evaluation of the upper gastrointestinal tract is required.

Endoscopic (eg, esophagogastroduodenoscopy, colonoscopy, enteroscopy, or capsule endoscopy) or radiographic (eg, barium enema, upper

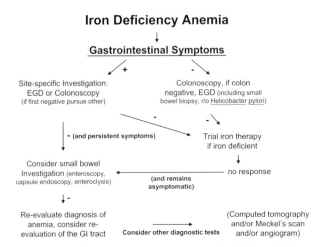

Fig. 2. Algorithm for evaluation of patients with iron deficiency anemia. Although the management of each patient with iron deficiency anemia should be individualized, several general points are worthy of emphasis. First, evaluation should begin with clear documentation of an iron deficiency state. The proposed algorithm indicates that gastrointestinal tract studies initially should be based on history and physical examination, in particular with gastrointestinal symptoms in mind. In the asymptomatic patient with a negative colon exam and unremarkable upper gastrointestinal tract exam, celiac disease must be considered, and small bowel biopsy is recommended for most patients. For evaluation of the small bowel, several options are available; it is unknown which is superior. This algorithm does not incorporate recommendations for premenopausal women, who are more difficult to assess and manage because of confounding menstrual blood loss. (*From* Rockey DC. Gastrointestinal bleeding. In: Feldman M, Friedman LS, Sleisenger MH, editors. Sleisenger & Fordtran's gastrointestinal and liver disease. 7th edition. Philadelphia: Saunders; 2002. p. 211–48; with permission.)

gastrointestinal series, enteroclysis, CT, or computed tomographic colonography) tests have been used to evaluate the gastrointestinal tract in patients who have iron deficiency anemia. Radiographic studies are effective for detecting masses and large ulcerating lesions throughout the gastrointestinal tract [23]. Radiographic studies are typically not reliable for detection of mucosal lesions. Recently, computed tomographic colonography has been introduced as an alternative method to evaluate the colon [24–26]. Considerable controversy exists as to which style of test (ie, upper gastrointestinal series with or without small bowel follow-through, esophagogastroduodenoscopy, colonoscopy, enteroscopy, enteroclysis, capsule endoscopy in the upper gastrointestinal tract and air contrast barium enema, computed tomographic colonography, or colonoscopy in the lower gastrointestinal tract) is most appropriate. Each of these tests has a role. For example, if a mucosal lesion is suspected, an endoscopic approach is preferable. If on the other hand, a patient has risk factors that make endoscopy unsafe, radiographic tests are preferable. An important advantage of endoscopy in patients who have iron deficiency anemia is that from a practical standpoint, patients can be prepared to undergo both lower and upper examinations sequentially on one same day; for patients to undergo two barium procedures of the gastrointestinal tract, they would have to undergo separate preparation procedures and return on 2 separate days.

The small intestine is important to consider as a potential site of bleeding in patients with have negative examinations of the colon and upper gastrointestinal tract. Numerous approaches can be used to examine the small intestine. Radiographic examination of the small bowel (enteroclysis remains the best radiographic imaging modality for the small bowel) has been found to be of limited value in patients who have iron deficiency anemia and for the most part is not recommended [4]. Small bowel follow-through to examine the small bowel is particularly insensitive and is not recommended. In contrast, endoscopic evaluation of the small intestine has a greater sensitivity for mucosal abnormalities and possibly for mass lesions also; therefore, it has been advocated in patients who have negative colonic and upper gastrointestinal tract evaluations.

Endoscopy of the small intestine has undergone major changes over the last decade. Enteroscopy is usually of the push or sonde variety. Push enteroscopy consists of insertion of a long endoscope, usually a specialized enteroscope, it and should be the initial approach in most patients. Using conscious sedation, the enteroscope can be passed 50 to 60 cm beyond the ligament of Trietz, allowing examination of the distal duodenum and proximal jejunum. Push enteroscopy has been reported to identify a source of bleeding in from 6% to 27% of patients [27–29]. The major advantages of push enteroscopy are that it is readily available and relatively safe. Most importantly, biopsy and endoscopic therapy can be performed. Sonde enteroscopy is considerably more complex than push enteroscopy, involving placement of a long, small-caliber endoscope into the proximal small bowel; subsequent peristalsis carries the endoscope to the terminal ileum or even colon, permitting visualization of a large portion (or all) of the small bowel. Sonde enteroscopy essentially has been replaced by capsule endoscopy, and it is used by very few institutions. A new enteroscope, the double balloon enteroscope, allows deeper insertion into the small bowel [30,31]. Experience with it in patients who have iron deficiency anemia is limited. Intraoperative enteroscopy permits visualization of most or all of the small intestine with an enteroscope (or standard colonoscope), which is advanced manually through the small bowel by the surgeon during laparotomy. In patients who have iron deficiency anemia, it should be reserved for select (severe and medically unresponsive) cases.

The newest technology in the area of small bowel imaging surrounds capsule endoscopy. This technique (see Carey and colleagues in this issue) is a major advance in small bowel investigation, is approximately 11 by 26 mm in size, and contains four light emitting diodes, a lens, a camera, two batteries, and a radiofrequency transmitter. The capsule obtains at least two images per second, transmitting this data to a recording device worn by the patient. The data subsequently are downloaded to a computer workstation loaded with software that allows images to be analyzed. Because of the capsule's small size, it passes through the gastrointestinal tract harmlessly in nearly all patients. Patients typically undergo preparation to clear the gastrointestinal tract. Capsule endoscopy has been used in patients who have iron deficiency anemia and has been demonstrated to identify the full gamut of important small bowel lesions, including vascular ectasias, ulcers, and mass lesions [32,33] (the articles by Lin and Rockey and Carey elsewhere in this issue have examples of the types of lesions detected by capsule endoscopy). Although such results are exciting, an important limitation of capsule endoscopy is its inability to administer therapy. Further study is required to understand the role of capsule endoscopy compared with enteroscopy for managing patients who have iron deficiency anemia.

A major unresolved issue with small bowel evaluation in patients who have iron deficiency anemia has to do with its clinical impact. Although all of the currently available techniques can identify abnormalities in a substantial proportion of patients who have iron deficiency anemia (and new diagnoses can be expected), the cost and benefit of their use remain unknown. Further, whether a small bowel study should be part of initial evaluation for all patients who have iron deficiency anemia (and negative colonic and esophagogastroduodenal evaluations) is unresolved. This author believes that small bowel investigation, whether enteroclysis, enteroscopy, or capsule endoscopy, should be reserved for patients who have specific symptoms or those who have negative upper and lower gastrointestinal tract evaluation not responding to usual replacement iron therapy and who do not have gastrointestinal tract lesions at the time of repeat endoscopy (see Fig. 2).

Other diagnostic approaches also may contribute. For example, abdominal CT has been shown to identify lesions that endoscopy has failed to detect, in particular neoplastic mass lesions [34]. CT, however, is insensitive for detecting mucosal lesions.

Special Situations

Celiac sprue, a relatively common bowel disorder, is an important cause of iron deficiency anemia and merits special consideration. It can lead not only to malabsorption of iron, but also to occult bleeding [35] and should be excluded carefully in patients who have iron deficiency anemia. Celiac sprue is particularly common in patients of Northern European descent and the elderly. Celiac disease is relatively uncommon in patients of African American or Asian background. A high index of suspicion often is required to make the diagnosis; therefore, small bowel biopsies should be obtained routinely in patients without another obvious cause of iron deficiency anemia.

Premenopausal women who have iron deficiency anemia represent a unique challenge. The available data suggest that a substantial proportion of premenopausal women who have iron deficiency anemia have underlying gastrointestinal tract lesions [36,37]. Lesions have been identified as commonly in the upper gastrointestinal tract as in the colon, and a surprisingly high proportion of lesions have been neoplastic [36,37]. Although these data are striking, the appropriate degree of investigation for most premenopausal women who have iron deficiency anemia is unknown at. The author believes that individual management depends on the clinical situation for each patient. For example, in those who have gastrointestinal symptoms, weight loss, fecal occult blood, or severe anemia, gastrointestinal tract evaluation is indicated. For asymptomatic women or those who have abnormal menses, gastrointestinal tract evaluation should be performed in the setting of any atypical features or in those whose menstrual blood loss appears to be out of proportion to the severity of their iron deficiency anemia.

A body of literature suggests *Helicobacter pylori*-associated gastritis is an important cause of iron deficiency anemia. The mechanism underlying iron deficiency anemia in patients who have *H pylori* associated gastritis is likely multifactorial. On one hand, *H pylori* gastritis in Yupik Eskimos appears to be associated with substantial gastrointestinal tract bleeding [38]. On the other hand, it appears that *H pylori* gastritis may be associated with impaired iron absorption [39]. In either case, *H pylori* gastritis should be considered in all patients who have iron deficiency anemia.

Many patients who have iron deficiency anemia have no identifiable gastrointestinal tract abnormality after appropriate gastrointestinal evaluation. In this circumstance, explanations for iron deficiency anemia include non-gastrointestinal blood loss, misdiagnosis of the type of anemia, missed lesions, or nutritional deficiency. For these patients, it is imperative to exclude the possibility of extragastrointestinal blood loss and to verify that the anemia is caused by iron deficiency. A missed lesion must be considered in all of these patients; up to 25% of patients who have been found to have a negative colonoscopy and esophagogastroduodenoscopy are found to have upper gastrointestinal tract lesions at the time of repeat esophagogastroduodenoscopy [27,29,40]. It is particularly important to consider unusual and difficult-to-recognize lesions such Cameron lesions within a hiatal hernia, watermelon stomach, portal hypertensive gastropathy, and vascular ectasias. Colonoscopy also can miss important lesions. Therefore, repeat study of the gastrointestinal tract should be considered in patients who have persistent iron deficiency anemia despite iron repletion.

Another important possibility in patients who have unremarkable gastrointestinal tract evaluation is iron malabsorption. Clinically useful methods to precisely measure iron absorption are lacking, so further investigation is required in this area. Still, some data suggest that iron malabsorption could be important in patients who have iron deficiency anemia. One study found that approximately 20% of patients who have iron deficiency anemia and no obvious source of gastrointestinal tract lesion (documented by esophagogastroduodenoscopy and colonoscopy) had plasma gastrin levels above 200 ng/L, consistent with gastric achlorhydria [41]. All of these patients had gastric atrophy at the time of biopsy, and antibodies to gastric parietal cells or intrinsic factor were positive in most. Although fecal blood loss was not quantitated, all patients had negative fecal occult blood tests. These data imply that some patients who do not have gastrointestinal lesions could have iron malabsorption as a result of atrophic gastritis [41].

The prevalence and significance of iron deficiency without anemia requires further investigation, but recent data suggest that iron deficiency without anemia may be associated with significant gastrointestinal tract pathology [15,18].

Treatment and Outcome

Once the diagnosis of iron deficiency anemia has been confirmed, iron therapy should be instituted. Oral ferrous sulfate is recommended, because it is inexpensive and effective (the recommended dose is 300 mg three times daily). In those who are intolerant to ferrous sulfate, ferrous gluconate or fumarate are acceptable alternatives. Parenteral iron therapy should be used only for patients who have severe malabsorption or who are intolerant to iron supplements.

Specific management of patients who have iron deficiency anemia (and fecal occult blood) depends on the underlying disorder responsible for bleeding. Most mass lesions require surgical excision, although ulcerative processes usually can be managed with medical therapy. If patients are taking nonsteroidal anti-inflammatory drugs (NSAIDs), these should be discontinued, even if a lesion cannot be identified. The prognosis for patients who have iron deficiency anemia and lesions amenable to medical therapy (ie, duodenal ulcer, esophagitis, or large adenoma) is excellent.

Perhaps the most challenging patients are those who have vascular ectasias; these lesions are usually multiple, may be difficult to identify, and bleed recurrently, making management difficult. In addition, treatment of one does not preclude bleeding from another. Treatment of vascular ectasias is difficult, because they rarely are found in isolation. Patients who have lesions that are readily identified are best treated endoscopically with some form of thermal-based treatment (laser, bipolar electrocoagulation, bicap, or argon plasma coagulation), banding, or injection therapy; each of these techniques appears to be effective and relatively safe. Caution is urged, especially in the right colon because of the risk of perforation. For diffuse ectasias, the use of pharmacologic therapy with estrogen/progesterone compounds is controversial. These agents are thought to enhance clotting, although the mechanism is unknown [42,43]. In a prospective longitudinal observational study of 43 patients with proven or presumed vascular ectasias treated with Ortho-Novum 1/50, containing 1 mg of norethindrone and 0.05 mg of mestranol (one tablet twice daily) bleeding was halted. Adverse effects can be problematic, and include breast tenderness and vaginal bleeding in women and gynecomastia and loss of libido in men. Controlled trials using estrogen/progesterone compounds have failed to show an advantage over placebo [44,45]. Octreotide also has been tried in patients with bleeding caused by diffuse vascular ectasia. At a dose of 0.05 to 1 mg/d subcutaneously, this compound was reported to be effective and without adverse effects [46]. Unfortunately, carefully controlled trials are not available. Other agents, including aminocaproic acid, tranexamic acid, and danazol may be helpful, but again, controlled data are not available. The use of hormonal therapy is controversial.

The prognosis for patients who do not have lesions identified during gastrointestinal evaluation is favorable; very few are found to have significant gastrointestinal lesions at a later date. Most patients who have iron deficiency anemia and no identifiable gastrointestinal tract lesion respond to standard oral iron therapy. For patients who do not respond to iron therapy, the diagnosis of iron deficiency anemia should be re-evaluated, and repeat gastrointestinal evaluation should remain an important consideration.

FECAL OCCULT BLOOD

Fecal occult blood is the most common form of occult gastrointestinal bleeding. When fecal occult blood tests have been employed in large populations, 2% to 16% of those tested were positive [47–50]. Numerous different types of fecal occult blood tests are available. They are most commonly used to screen the colon for cancer [47,48,50], and in this setting, they have been shown to reduce mortality from colon cancer [47,48,50].

Fecal blood loss in normal individuals varies from 0.5 to 1.5 mL per day; most fecal occult blood tests begin to become positive at a level of around 2 mL of blood loss per day. Importantly, however, for fecal occult blood tests to become consistently positive, higher levels of fecal blood are required. The likelihood of detecting fecal blood depends on the type of fecal occult blood test used and individual characteristics, including the frequency with which the bleeding lesion bleeds, bowel motility, and the anatomic level of bleeding.

Fecal Occult Blood Tests

Fecal occult blood tests are capable of detecting blood from many different lesions at various levels in the gastrointestinal tract. In addition, the type of fecal occult blood test used determines from where in the gastrointestinal tract blood is most likely to be detected (Table 3). When considering the different types of fecal occult blood tests, an understanding of intraluminal metabolism of hemoglobin is critical (Fig. 3).

Guaiac-based tests

The classic fecal occult blood test has been of the guaiac-based type (see Table 3). Guaiac-based tests take advantage of the fact that hemoglobin possesses pseudoperoxidase activity; guaiac turns blue after oxidation by oxidants or peroxidases in the presence of an oxygen donor such as hydrogen peroxide. Guaiac tests are more sensitive for detecting bleeding from the lower than upper gastrointestinal tract, because hemoglobin is degraded in the gastrointestinal tract (see Fig. 3). The characteristics of specific guaiac-based tests vary. For example, of the two most commonly used tests in the United States, Hemoccult II and Hemoccult II SENSA (both from SmithKline Diagnostics, Palo Alto, California), the latter is substantially more sensitive for detecting fecal heme than the former [51,52]. This is important, because the more sensitive a test is for detection of fecal blood, the lower the specificity for detection of colon cancer.

Table 3
Characteristics of fecal occult blood tests

Variable	Guaiac	Heme-Porphyrin	Immunochemical
Detection characteristics			
Upper gastrointestinal	+	++++	0
Small bowel	++	++++	+
Right colonic	+++	++++	+++
Left colonic	++++	++++	++++
Test factors			
Bedside availability	++++	0	+
Time to develop	1 minute	1 hour	5 min to 24
False positives			
Animal hemoglobin	++++	++++	0
Dietary peroxidases	+++	0	0
False negatives			
Hemoglobin degradation	++	0	++
Storage	++	++++	++
Vitamin C	++	0	0

Relative comparisons are shown on a scale of 0 to ++++, with 0 being the negative and ++++ being highly positive.

Adapted from Rockey DC. Occult gastrointestinal bleeding. N Engl J Med 1999;341:38–46. © 1999 Massachusetts Medical Society. All rights reserved; with permission.

At the same time, highly sensitive based tests are more likely to detect blood from the upper gastrointestinal tract and small intestine.

The likelihood that a guaiac-based test will be positive (ie, that it will detect fecal heme) is related to the quantity of blood present in the stool, which in turn is related to the size and location of the bleeding lesion [53,54]. Because bleeding colon lesions are more likely to lead to undegraded blood and heme in the stool, guaiac-based tests are best at detecting such distal lesions. Other factors, however, such as stool transit time, stool mixing, and whether there has been intraluminal degradation of heme, are important and likely account for the substantial variability in the content of fecal hemoglobin [55]. It appears that fecal hemoglobin levels must exceed 10 mg/g (10 mL daily blood loss) before Hemoccult II tests are positive at least 50% of the time [56]. On the other hand, stools containing less than 1 mg/g hemoglobin may result in a positive guaiac-based test in certain situations.

It is also important to emphasize that various factors influence guaiac test results. For example, fecal rehydration affects the reactivity of guaiac-based tests; it raises sensitivity but reduces specificity [50]. Additionally, diet is important (see Table 3), because foods that contain peroxidases can cause positive guaiac test results. It is believed that oral iron causes positive guaiac tests. The dark-green or black appearance of iron in stool, however, should not be confused with the blue typical of a positive guaiac reaction; indeed, prospective studies have demonstrated that orally administered iron, even in large amounts, does not cause a positive guaiac reaction [57]. Finally, bismuth-containing

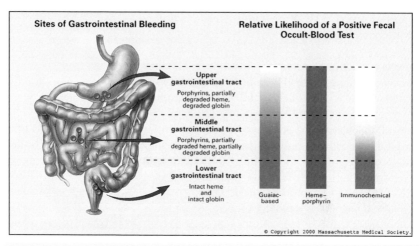

Fig. 3. Sites of gastrointestinal bleeding, intraluminal metabolism of hemoglobin, and detection of intraluminal blood by fecal occult blood tests. Hemoglobin is cleaved to heme and globin by gastric pepsin or pancreatic proteases in the upper gastrointestinal tract. Heme that is not absorbed is converted to porphyrins and iron by poorly understood mechanisms. This fraction is not detected by guaiac tests but is detected by the heme-porphyrin assay (HemoQuant), which measures both heme and porphyrins, and is therefore a highly accurate indicator of bleeding, regardless of level. Globin in the upper gastrointestinal tract is digested by pepsin, pancreatic, and intestinal proteases and thus is not detected by immunochemical fecal occult blood tests. (*From* Rockey DC. Occult gastrointestinal bleeding. N Engl J Med 1999;341:38–46. © 1999 Massachusetts Medical Society. All rights reserved; with permission.)

antacids and antidiarrheals cause the stool to be dark and should not be confused with a positive guaiac reaction.

Immunochemical-based tests

Immunochemical fecal occult blood tests (see Table 3) detect human globin epitopes and are highly sensitive for detection of blood [58]. Further, they do not detect blood from upper gastrointestinal sources (see Fig. 3), because globin molecules are degraded by enzymes found in the upper gastrointestinal tract. Therefore, they have a theoretical advantage over guaiac-based tests in terms of specificity for detection of colonic lesions. They are limited, however, by technical problems such as loss of hemoglobin antigenicity at room temperature and the general requirement for more intensive laboratory processing.

Heme-porphyrin based tests

The heme-porphyrin test (HemoQuant, Mayo Medical Laboratories, Rochester, Minnesota) relies on a spectrofluorometric method to measure porphyrin derived from heme, and therefore provides a highly accurate determination of total stool hemoglobin (see Table 3). Although neither intraluminal degradation of hemoglobin nor interfering peroxidase producing substances affect the heme-porphyrin assay, an important problem with this test is myoglobin, a heme-containing protein found in red meats that is measured as heme-porphyrin. The heme-porphyrin test is the most sensitive method of detecting occult blood loss.

Differential Diagnosis and Approach to Evaluation

The history and physical examination can provide information important to the clinician when considering differential diagnosis. As for iron deficiency anemia, the focus first should be on gastrointestinal symptoms. Additionally, a history of medications that can injure the gastrointestinal mucosa, including NSAIDs, alendronate, and potassium chloride should be sought. Use of anticoagulants is also important. A family history of bleeding should be sought (ie, hereditary hemorrhagic telangiectasia). Signs are also important, and may signify underlying systemic disorders. Many systemic disorders have cutaneous manifestations and should be considered during the physical examination. For example, patients with occult bleeding caused by celiac sprue may have dermatitis herpetiformis. Neurofibromas, cafe au lait spots, and axillary freckles are found in patients with neurofibromatosis. The polyposis syndromes (Peutz-Jeghers syndrome, Gardner syndrome, and Cronkite-Canada syndrome) often have cutaneous abnormalities.

As with iron deficiency anemia, essentially any gastrointestinal lesion can lead to occult bleeding and positive fecal occult blood tests, including lesions that often are associated with acute bleeding. Lesions most commonly responsible for occult bleeding are highlighted in Table 1. Although the colon traditionally has been considered to be the source of most occult gastrointestinal blood loss, the upper gastrointestinal tract is also a prominent cause of occult bleeding. The most common causes of fecal occult blood include colon adenocarcinoma, large colonic adenomatous polyps (greater than 2 cm) gastroduodenal ulcers, vascular ectasias, esophagitis, and gastritis. Less common, but important causes of occult bleeding include various small intestinal lesions (tumors, ulcers), upper gastrointestinal mass lesions (adenocarcinoma, adenomas), gastric vascular ectasia, and Cameron lesions.

In asymptomatic patients found to have occult blood in the stool, investigation initially should be focused on the colon (Fig. 4). Colonoscopy and air contrast barium enema are the most commonly used tests, although there is controversy with regard to which is the most appropriate investigative modality. It is recommended that flexible sigmoidoscopy be used in combination with air contrast barium enema so that the recto–sigmoid colon is evaluated fully, although new data suggest that air contrast barium enema is as accurate in the left colon as it is in the right colon [59]. Recently, computed tomographic colonography has been introduced as an alternative method to evaluate the colon [25,26]. The test chosen by the provider (and patient) to evaluate the colon for fecal blood likely will vary, and depends on local expertise, comfort of the patient with a specific test, and test availability.

In patients who have gastrointestinal symptoms that suggest specific diagnoses (ie, change in stool caliber, epigastric pain, or heartburn) initial investigation should be directed toward the location of specific symptoms (see Fig. 4).

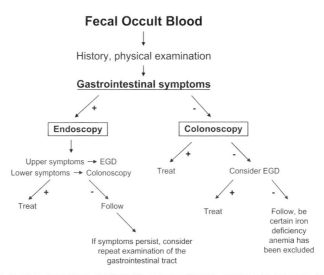

Fig. 4. Algorithm for evaluation of patients with fecal occult blood. As with iron deficiency anemia, the approach to fecal occult blood should begin with a careful history and physical examination. Most patients should undergo colonoscopy initially. In the patient who has clear upper gastrointestinal symptoms, esophagogastroduodenoscopy should be considered initially. In the asymptomatic patient with a negative colon exam, evaluation of the upper gastrointestinal tract should be considered. EGD, esophagogastroduodenoscopy.

Synchronous lesions are rare, and identification of an abnormality clearly consistent with bleeding such as a large mass lesion, large ulceration, or severe inflammation means that further evaluation (ie, of the remaining gastrointestinal tract) is probably not necessary.

The upper gastrointestinal tract is an important potential source of bleeding in patients with fecal occult blood but a normal colonic examination. In studies that have addressed this issue, potential bleeding sites have been identified frequently in the upper gastrointestinal tract (Fig. 5) [36,60–64]. Not only did investigation with endoscopy lead to the finding of upper gastrointestinal tract malignancies in all of the studies examining these patients, but it also led to management changes in a high proportion of patients. The finding of upper gastrointestinal lesions in patients who have positive guaiac-based tests (such as those used in these reports) may be considered somewhat surprising, because this type of test is thought to have a relatively low sensitivity for detecting upper gastrointestinal blood. Guaiac-based tests, however, particularly the more sensitive tests, are capable of detecting small amounts of upper gastrointestinal tract blood [52]. Further, many of the types of lesions identified in the upper gastrointestinal tract in these studies bleed enough to produce positive guaiac-based tests [6,65]. A major question, however, remains, and surrounds the question of whether it is cost-effective to perform with upper

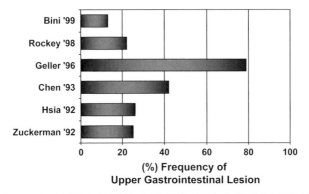

Fig. 5. Prevalence of upper gastrointestinal tract abnormalities in patients with fecal occult blood and negative colon examination. Study authors of investigations focused on upper gastro-intestinal tract evaluation in patients with fecal occult blood, and negative colon exams are shown. Definition of an upper gastrointestinal lesion varied among studies, but in general, lesions that were felt to be consistent with occult gastrointestinal bleeding were considered upper gastrointestinal lesions. The number of patients in enrolled in the studies ranged from 53 to 498.

gastrointestinal tract investigation in patients who have fecal occult blood and a normal colonic examination.

The appropriate evaluation for patients with fecal occult blood detected at the time of digital rectal examination remains controversial. Anorectal trauma or dietary factors in this setting may lead to false-positive tests. In both symptomatic and asymptomatic patients with fecal occult blood detected by digital rectal examination, however, the number of new lesions identified by gastrointestinal evaluation is substantial [63,66,67]. In fact, available data suggest that the diagnostic yield given occult blood detected by digital rectal examination is similar if not greater than that detected in spontaneously passed stools [63,67]. Thus, the available data suggest that evaluation is warranted.

Occult gastrointestinal bleeding often is ascribed to anticoagulant or aspirin therapy. It has been demonstrated, however, that fecal blood levels in patients therapeutically anticoagulated appeared to be normal [68,69]. Low-dose aspirin alone resulted in only small elevations in fecal blood levels, while the combination of aspirin and warfarin caused slightly higher elevations in fecal blood levels [68,69]. Neither warfarin nor low-dose aspirin alone appear to cause positive guaiac-based fecal occult blood tests [69]. Thus, a positive fecal occult blood test should not be considered to be caused by anticoagulation or aspirin alone. Rather, a positive fecal occult blood test should raise the possibility of a gastrointestinal tract abnormality and thus should lead to appropriate evaluation. In a prospective study evaluating the gastrointestinal tract in anticoagulated patients with positive guaiac-based fecal occult blood tests, 15 of 16 had previously undiagnosed lesions, 20% of which were malignant [70].

Treatment

As with iron deficiency anemia, management of patients with fecal occult blood depends on the underlying etiology of bleeding. General recommendations for management are as for iron deficiency anemia. The prognosis of patients with positive fecal occult blood tests but no identifiable gastrointestinal pathology appears to be favorable, but this has not been studied rigorously.

SUMMARY

Occult gastrointestinal bleeding commonly manifests as iron deficiency anemia or fecal occult blood. Iron deficiency anemia results from chronic occult gastrointestinal bleeding. Evaluation of asymptomatic patients who have iron deficiency anemia or fecal occult blood usually should begin with investigation of the colon. Colonoscopy is preferred, but flexible sigmoidoscopy plus air contrast barium enema, or computed tomographic colonography may be acceptable in certain circumstances. If evaluation of the colon does not reveal a bleeding site, evaluation of the upper gastrointestinal tract is mandatory in patients who have iron deficiency anemia, and this should be considered in those who have fecal occult blood. In patients who have gastrointestinal symptoms, evaluation of the portion of the gastrointestinal tract from which the symptoms is derived should be pursued initially. The role of small intestinal investigation is controversial, and this probably should be reserved for patients who have iron deficiency anemia and persistent gastrointestinal symptoms or those who fail to respond to appropriate therapy. Celiac sprue should be considered as a potential cause of iron deficiency anemia in all patients. The treatment and prognosis of patients who have iron deficiency anemia or fecal occult blood depends on the gastrointestinal tract abnormality(ies) identified. Those without identifiable bleeding sites generally respond to conservative management and have a favorable prognosis. On the other hand, the outlook is poorer for patients with refractory occult blood loss or those who have vascular ectasias. Both groups of patients are clinically challenging and require a focused and experienced team approach to diagnosis and therapy.

References

[1] Schiff L, Stevens RJ, Shapiro N, et al. Observations on the oral administration of citrate blood in man. Am J Med Sci 1942;203:409.

[2] Looker AC, Dallman PR, Carroll MD, et al. Prevalence of iron deficiency in the United States. JAMA 1997;277:973.

[3] Hallberg L, Hogdahl AM, Nilsson L, et al. Menstrual blood loss and iron deficiency. Acta Med Scand 1966;180:639.

[4] Rockey DC. Occult gastrointestinal bleeding. N Engl J Med 1999;341:38.

[5] Hentze MW, Muckenthaler MU, Andrews NC. Balancing acts: molecular control of mammalian iron metabolism. Cell 2004;117:285.

[6] Ahlquist DA, McGill DB, Schwartz S, et al. Fecal blood levels in health and disease. A study using HemoQuant. N Engl J Med 1985;312:1422.

[7] Dybdahl JH, Daae LN, Larsen S. Occult faecal blood loss determined by chemical tests and a 51 Cr method. Scand J Gastroenterol 1981;16:245.

[8] Massey AC. Microcytic anemia. Differential diagnosis and management of iron deficiency anemia. Med Clin North Am 1992;76:549.

[9] Cook IJ, Pavli P, Riley JW, et al. Gastrointestinal investigation of iron deficiency anemia. BMJ 1986;292:1380.

[10] Gordon S, Bensen S, Smith R. Long-term follow-up of older patients with iron deficiency anemia after a negative GI evaluation. Am J Gastroenterol 1996;91:885.

[11] Gordon SR, Smith RE, Power GC. The role of endoscopy in the evaluation of iron deficiency anemia in patients over the age of 50. Am J Gastroenterol 1994;89:1963.

[12] Gostout CJ. Enteroscopy for unexplained iron-deficiency anemia: identifying the patient with sprue. Gastrointest Endosc 1993;39:76.

[13] Ho CH, Chau WK, Hsu HC, et al. Predictive risk factors and prevalence of malignancy in patients with iron deficiency anemia in Taiwan. Am J Hematol 2005;78:108.

[14] Kepczyk T, Kadakia SC. Prospective evaluation of gastrointestinal tract in patients with iron-deficiency anemia. Dig Dis Sci 1995;40:1283.

[15] Lee JG, Sahagun G, Oehlke M, et al. Serious gastrointestinal pathology found in patients with serum ferritin values < 50 ng/ml. Am J Gastroenterol 1998;93:772.

[16] McIntyre AS, Long RG. Prospective survey of investigations in outpatients referred with iron deficiency anaemia. Gut 1993;34:1102.

[17] Rockey DC, Cello JP. Evaluation of the gastrointestinal tract in patients with iron-deficiency anemia. N Engl J Med 1993;329:1691.

[18] Wilcox CM, Alexander LN, Clark WS. Prospective evaluation of the gastrointestinal tract in patients with iron deficiency and no systemic or gastrointestinal symptoms or signs. Am J Med 1997;103:405.

[19] St John DJ, Young GP. Evaluation of radiochromium blood loss studies in unexplained iron-deficiency anaemia. Aust N Z J Med 1978;8:121.

[20] Ferguson A, Brydon WG, Brian H, et al. Use of whole gut perfusion to investigate gastrointestinal blood loss in patients with iron deficiency anaemia. Gut 1996;38:120.

[21] Niv E, Elis A, Zissin R, et al. Iron deficiency anemia in patients without gastrointestinal symptoms—a prospective study. Fam Pract 2005;22:58.

[22] Capurso G, Baccini F, Osborn J, et al. Can patient characteristics predict the outcome of endoscopic evaluation of iron deficiency anemia: a multiple logistic regression analysis. Gastrointest Endosc 2004;59:766.

[23] Ott DJ, Gelfand DW. The future of barium radiology. Br J Radiol 1997;70:S171.

[24] Dachman AH, Yoshida H. Virtual colonoscopy: past, present, and future. Radiol Clin North Am 2003;41:377.

[25] Rockey DC. Colon imaging: computed tomographic colonography. Clin Gastroenterol Hepatol 2005;3:S37.

[26] Van Dam J, Cotton P, Johnson CD, et al. AGA future trends report: CT colonography. Gastroenterology 2004;127:970.

[27] Chak A, Cooper GS, Canto MI, et al. Enteroscopy for the initial evaluation of iron deficiency. Gastrointest Endosc 1998;47:144.

[28] Eisen GM, Dominitz JA, Faigel DO, et al. Enteroscopy. Gastrointest Endosc 2001;53:871.

[29] Landi B, Tkoub M, Gaudric M, et al. Diagnostic yield of push-type enteroscopy in relation to indication. Gut 1998;42:421.

[30] May A, Nachbar L, Ell C. Double-balloon enteroscopy (push-and-pull enteroscopy) of the small bowel: feasibility and diagnostic and therapeutic yield in patients with suspected small bowel disease. Gastrointest Endosc 2005;62:62.

[31] Yamamoto H, Yano T, Kita H, et al. New system of double-balloon enteroscopy for diagnosis and treatment of small intestinal disorders. Gastroenterology 2003;125:1556.

[32] Bar-Meir S, Eliakim R, Nadler M, et al. Second capsule endoscopy for patients with severe iron deficiency anemia. Gastrointest Endosc 2004;60:711.

[33] Pennazio M, Santucci R, Rondonotti E, et al. Outcome of patients with obscure gastrointestinal bleeding after capsule endoscopy: report of 100 consecutive cases. Gastroenterology 2004;126:643.
[34] Niv E, Elis A, Zissin R, et al. Abdominal computed tomography in the evaluation of patients with asymptomatic iron deficiency anemia: a prospective study. Am J Med 2004;117:193.
[35] Fine KD. The prevalence of occult gastrointestinal bleeding in celiac sprue. N Engl J Med 1996;334:1163.
[36] Bini EJ, Rajapaksa RC, Valdes MT, et al. Is upper gastrointestinal endoscopy indicated in asymptomatic patients with a positive fecal occult blood test and negative colonoscopy? Am J Med 1999;106:613.
[37] Green BT, Rockey DC. Gastrointestinal endoscopic evaluation of premenopausal women with iron deficiency anemia. J Clin Gastroenterol 2004;38:104.
[38] Yip R, Limburg PJ, Ahlquist DA, et al. Pervasive occult gastrointestinal bleeding in an Alaska native population with prevalent iron deficiency. Role of Helicobacter pylori gastritis. JAMA 1997;277:1135.
[39] Annibale B, Capurso G, Lahner E, et al. Concomitant alterations in intragastric pH and ascorbic acid concentration in patients with Helicobacter pylori gastritis and associated iron deficiency anaemia. Gut 2003;52:496.
[40] Zaman A, Katon RM. Puch enteroscopy for obscure gastrointestinal bleeding yields a high incidence of proximal lesions within reach of a standard endoscope. Gastrointest Endosc 1998;47:372.
[41] Dickey W, Kenny BD, McMillan SA, et al. Gastric as well as duodenal biopsies may be useful in the investigation of iron deficiency anaemia. Scand J Gastroenterol 1997;32:469.
[42] Barkin JS, Ross BS. Medical therapy for chronic gastrointestinal bleeding of obscure origin. Am J Gastroenterol 1998;93:1250.
[43] van Cutsem E, Rutgeerts P, Vantrappen G. Treatment of bleeding gastrointestinal vascular malformations with oestrogen-progesterone. Lancet 1990;335:953.
[44] Junquera F, Feu F, Papo M, et al. A multicenter, randomized, clinical trial of hormonal therapy in the prevention of rebleeding from gastrointestinal angiodysplasia. Gastroenterology 2001;121:1073.
[45] Lewis BS, Salomon P, Rivera-MacMurray S, et al. Does hormonal therapy have any benefit for bleeding angiodysplasia? J Clin Gastroenterol 1992;15:99.
[46] Nardone G, Rocco A, Balzano T, et al. The efficacy of octreotide therapy in chronic bleeding due to vascular abnormalities of the gastrointestinal tract. Aliment Pharmacol Ther 1999;13:1429.
[47] Hardcastle JD, Chamberlain J, Robinson MHE, et al. Randomised controlled trial of faecal-occult-blood screening for colorectal cancer. Lancet 1996;348:1472.
[48] Kronborg O, Fenger C, Olsen J, et al. Randomised study of screening for colorectal cancer with faecal-occult-blood test. Lancet 1996;348:1467.
[49] Levin B, Hess K, Johnson C. Screening for colorectal cancer. A comparison of 3 fecal occult blood tests. Arch Intern Med 1997;157:970.
[50] Mandel JS, Bond JH, Church TR, et al. Reducing mortality from colorectal cancer by screening for fecal occult blood. Minnesota Colon Cancer Control Study. [published erratum appears in N Engl J Med 1993;329(9):672] [see comments]. N Engl J Med 1993;328:1365.
[51] Allison JE, Tekawa IS, Ransom LJ, et al. A comparison of fecal occult-blood tests for colorectal-cancer screening. N Engl J Med 1996;334:155.
[52] Rockey DC, Auslander A, Greenberg PD. Detection of upper gastrointestinal blood with fecal occult blood tests. Am J Gastroenterol 1999;94:344.
[53] Dybdahl JH, Daae LN, Larsen S, et al. Occult faecal blood loss determined by a 51Cr method and chemical tests in patients referred for colonoscopy. Scand J Gastroenterol 1984;19:245.

[54] Herzog P, Holtermuller KH, Preiss J, et al. Fecal blood loss in patients with colonic polyps: a comparison of measurements with 51chromium-labeled erythrocytes and with the Haemoccult test. Gastroenterology 1982;83:957.

[55] Ahlquist DA, McGill DB, Fleming JL, et al. Patterns of occult bleeding in asymptomatic colorectal cancer. Cancer 1989;63:1826.

[56] Stroehlein JR, Fairbanks VF, McGill DB, et al. Hemoccult detection of fecal occult blood quantitated by radioassay. Am J Dig Dis 1976;21:841.

[57] Laine LA, Bentley E, Chandrasoma P. Effect of oral iron therapy on the upper gastrointestinal tract. A prospective evaluation. Dig Dis Sci 1988;33:172.

[58] Saito H. Screening for colorectal cancer by immunochemical fecal occult blood testing. Jpn J Cancer Res 1996;87:1011.

[59] Thompson WT, Paulson E, Rockey DC. Causes of errors in polyp detection on air contrast barium enema. Radiology, in press.

[60] Chen YK, Gladden DR, Kestenbaum DJ, et al. Is there a role for upper gastrointestinal endoscopy in the evaluation of patients with occult blood-positive stool and negative colonoscopy? Am J Gastroenterol 1993;88:2026.

[61] Geller AJ, Kolts BE, Achem SR, et al. The high frequency of upper gastrointestinal pathology in patients with fecal occult blood and colon polyps. Am J Gastroenterol 1993;88:1184.

[62] Hsia PC, al-Kawas FH. Yield of upper endoscopy in the evaluation of asymptomatic patients with Hemoccult-positive stool after a negative colonoscopy. Am J Gastroenterol 1992;87:1571.

[63] Rockey DC, Koch J, Cello JP, et al. Relative frequency of upper gastrointestinal and colonic lesions in patients with positive fecal occult-blood tests. N Engl J Med 1998;339:153.

[64] Zuckerman G, Benitez J. A prospective study of bidirectional endoscopy (colonoscopy and upper endoscopy) in the evaluation of patients with occult gastrointestinal bleeding. Am J Gastroenterol 1992;87:62.

[65] Dybdahl JH. Occult faecal blood loss determined by a 51Cr method and chemical tests in patients referred for upper gastrointestinal endoscopy. Scand J Gastroenterol 1984;19:235.

[66] Bini EJ, Rajapaksa RC, Weinshel EH. The findings and impact of nonrehydrated guaiac examination of the rectum (FINGER) study: a comparison of 2 methods of screening for colorectal cancer in asymptomatic average-risk patients. Arch Intern Med 1999;159:2022.

[67] Eisner MS, Lewis JH. Diagnostic yield of a positive fecal occult blood test found on digital rectal examination. Does the finger count? Arch Intern Med 1991;151:2180.

[68] Blackshear JL, Baker VS, Holland A, et al. Fecal hemoglobin excretion in elderly patients with atrial fibrillation: combined aspirin and low-dose warfarin vs conventional warfarin therapy. Arch Intern Med 1996;156:658.

[69] Greenberg PD, Cello JP, Rockey DC. Asymptomatic chronic gastrointestinal blood loss in patients taking aspirin or warfarin for cardiovascular disease. Am J Med 1996;100:598.

[70] Jaffin BW, Bliss CM, LaMont JT. Significance of occult gastrointestinal bleeding during anticoagulation therapy. Am J Med 1987;83:269.

Gastroenterol Clin N Am 34 (2005) 719–734

GASTROENTEROLOGY CLINICS
OF NORTH AMERICA

ELSEVIER
SAUNDERS

Investigation of the Small Bowel in Gastrointestinal Bleeding—Enteroscopy and Capsule Endoscopy

Elizabeth J. Carey, MD, David E. Fleischer, MD*

Gastroenterology and Hepatology, Mayo Clinic, 13400 East Shea Boulevard, Scottsdale, AZ, USA

Small intestinal bleeding, or that which occurs between the ligament of Treitz and the ileocecal valve, represents a unique and challenging problem because of the small intestine's relative inaccessibility to traditional endoscopy. With the exception of the proximal duodenum and the distal ileum, upper and lower endoscopy do not visualize the small intestine. The length of the small intestine (approximately 14 feet) and its anatomic features (a loosely supported and looped structure on the mesentery) make conventional endoscopic techniques difficult and frequently inadequate.

Small intestinal bleeding presents a diagnostic challenge. Localization of the bleeding site cannot be guessed by the clinical history, as the patient may present with bright red or maroon blood per rectum, melena, or iron deficiency anemia. Causes of small intestinal bleeding are shown in Box 1. Upper or lower endoscopy, the usual initial evaluation of gastrointestinal (GI) bleeding, will be negative in the patient who has a small intestinal source. If bleeding continues, the patient meets the definition of obscure GI bleeding (OGIB), ongoing or recurrent intestinal bleeding without a cause found at original endoscopy. Small bowel bleeding comprises approximately 5% of OGIB [1].

Small intestinal bleeding presents a unique clinical problem that differs from upper and lower GI bleeding in many respects. Patients who have small intestinal bleeding undergo more diagnostic procedures, require more blood transfusions, have longer hospitalizations, and have higher health care expenditures than patients who have upper or lower GI bleeding[2]. The difficulty accessing the small bowel endoscopically may contribute to this phenomenon. Causes of

*Corresponding author. E-mail address: fleischer.david@mayo.edu (D.E. Fleischer).

0889-8553/05/$ – see front matter
doi:10.1016/j.gtc.2005.08.009

Box 1: Causes of small bowel bleeding

Angiodysplasia

Dieulafoy's lesions

Erosions/ulcers

Crohn's disease

Small bowel varices

Tumors

NSAID enteropathy

Radiation enteritis

Small bowel diverticulosis

Small bowel polyps

Aortoenteric fistula

Meckel's diverticulum

gastrointestinal bleeding that commonly are missed on upper endoscopy include:

- Cameron's erosions
- Gastric varices
- Dieulafoy's lesion
- Angiodysplasia
- Esophagitis
- Portal hypertensive gastropathy
- Gastric antral vascular ectasia

This article reviews pertinent enteroscopy techniques, with an emphasis on the new technologies of capsule endoscopy and double balloon enteroscopy.

ENTEROSCOPY

The field of small bowel enteroscopy has advanced tremendously over the past 30 years. Interested readers are referred to a review of the history of enteroscopy by Lewis [3]. Despite these advances, small bowel enteroscopy continues to be an evolving field, as gastroenterologists strive to minimize risk and patient discomfort while increasing the ability to diagnose and treat small bowel lesions.

Sonde Enteroscopy

Sonde enteroscopy largely has fallen out of favor and is now primarily of historical interest. Introduced in the mid-1980s, sonde enteroscopy marked the first successful efforts to reach past the middle small bowel. Sonde enteroscopy was performed with a long, thin (working length 270 to 280 cm, outer diameter 4.5 to 7.8 mm) enteroscope advanced through the small intestine by peristaltic action (Fig. 1). The sonde enteroscope was introduced transnasally and

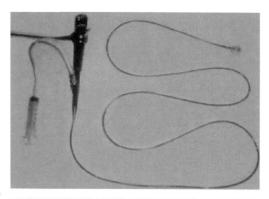

Fig. 1. Sonde enteroscope. (*Courtesy of* Blair Lewis, MD.)

advanced to the duodenum, where an air-filled balloon at the tip of the endoscope gripped the intestinal lumen. The balloon acted as a tractor against the intestinal wall, resulting in advancement of the endoscope by peristalsis. The instrument usually was placed in the morning, with the endoscopic examination occurring 6 to 8 hours later. Examination of the intestinal mucosa was performed upon withdrawal, which typically took 30 to 45 minutes [4].

Although sonde enteroscopy allowed for visualization of the entire small intestine, numerous limitations contributed to its demise. The sonde enteroscope lacked a deflectable tip and was not able to be advanced manually, limiting control of the investigator to examine areas of particular interest. Furthermore, the enteroscope did not have a working channel to allow for biopsy or therapeutic intervention. The procedure required up to 6 to 8 hours and was uncomfortable for the patient. For these reasons, enthusiasm waned, and the procedure is performed rarely now.

Push Enteroscopy

Push enteroscopy is probably the most commonly performed small bowel procedure today, as it often is pursued when upper endoscopy and colonoscopy have failed to find a source for blood loss. Push enteroscopy may be performed using dedicated enteroscopes or pediatric colonoscopes. Both are available with variable stiffness adjustments. Enteroscopes are significantly longer than colonoscopes (200 to 240 cm versus 135 cm), but the outer diameters are similar (about 11.5 mm), as are the internal channel diameters (3.2 to 3.8mm) (Fig. 2). Diagnostic and therapeutic options are comparable, but pediatric colonoscopes are more widely available in most settings.

Improving the depth of intubation into the small intestine is a frequently addressed topic in the literature. Depth of insertion is difficult to assess given the absence of anatomic landmarks in the small intestine. One method of estimation is to count the number of folds in the small intestine as the endoscope is withdrawn. This is labor-intensive and rarely practical. Fluoroscopy may aid in estimation but cannot provide exact localization. Even at the maximal depth

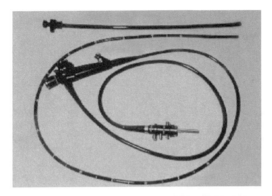

Fig. 2. Push enteroscope with overtube. (Courtesy of Blair Lewis, MD.)

of insertion, approximately 160 cm past the ligament of Treitz, over 250 cm of small intestine remains unexamined.

The use of an overtube to prevent looping of the instrument in the stomach increases insertion depth by 10 to 25 cm [5,6]. Many practitioners, however, have abandoned this practice, because overtubes contribute to reduced instrument mobility, increased patient discomfort, and increased complications. Mallory-Weiss tears, esophageal perforation, and pancreatitis (as a result of duodenal compression) [7] are reported complications related to overtube use during enteroscopy.

Prototype variable stiffness enteroscopes are emerging in an attempt to achieve maximal insertion depth without the use of an overtube [6,8]. In small studies, the variable stiffness enteroscopes achieve insertion depths comparable to a standard instrument with an overtube, but neither the diagnostic yield nor patient tolerance improves. Further research will help to determine how these enteroscopes will be integrated into clinical practice.

In patients who have OGIB, push enteroscopy is reported to find the bleeding lesion in 30% to 50% of cases [3]. The obvious limitation of push enteroscopy is the inability to reach lesions distal to the middle jejunum. In a series of 545 patients who underwent tandem push enteroscopy followed by sonde enteroscopy for GI bleeding, the yield for push enteroscopy was 41% compared with 65% in sonde enteroscopy [9]. A change in working diagnosis or management as a result of the findings on push enteroscopy occurs in 50% to 55% of cases [10,11].

One benefit of push enteroscopy is that it allows for a second-look at the esophagus, stomach, and proximal small bowel for lesions that may have been missed on original endoscopy. Indeed, 25% to 40% of lesions found on push enteroscopy are within reach of a standard gastroscope [9,12]. Another important benefit of push enteroscopy is the ability to provide diagnostic and therapeutic capabilities during one procedure. Biopsy, electrocautery, injection, and polypectomy are accomplished easily. Furthermore, push enteroscopy often can be performed in the outpatient setting without special equipment, making this procedure more widely available than other forms of enteroscopy.

Complications from push enteroscopy are infrequent, occurring in less than 1% of cases [9,13,14]. Most complications are related to use of an overtube, including Mallory-Weiss tear, pancreatitis (from duodenal compression), pharyngeal tear, and gastric mucosal stripping [15]. Because it is widely available, does not require additional endoscopist skill, and provides excellent visualization of the mucosa with therapeutic capability, push enteroscopy has been the workhorse of investigating the small bowel for bleeding.

Double Balloon Enteroscopy

The newest modality for imaging the small bowel was introduced in 2001, when Yamamoto and colleagues described their results using a double balloon method in four patients [16]. In the first three patients, an upper endoscope was able to reach 30 to 50 cm beyond the ligament of Treitz, and in the fourth patient, the ileocecal valve was reached using a longer enteroscope. Short of an intraoperative examination, double balloon enteroscopy represents the first successful achievement of providing both diagnostic and therapeutic intervention to the entire small bowel. Double balloon enteroscopy is unique in that it allows for visualization of the entire small intestine without advancing an excessive length of endoscope into the patient. The Fujinon double balloon video enteroscope (Fujinon, Inc., Wayne, New Jersey) has a working length of 200 cm, an outer diameter of 8.5 mm, and a working channel of 2.2 to 2.8 mm. The overtube is 140 cm in length, with an outer diameter of 12 mm. As inferred from its name, the two inflatable balloons are the crux of the double balloon system. The distal ends of the overtube and of the endoscope are fitted with inflatable/deflatable air-filled latex balloons (Fig. 3). When inflated to 45 mmHg, the balloons grip the intestinal lumen, providing traction against the wall without undue pressure.

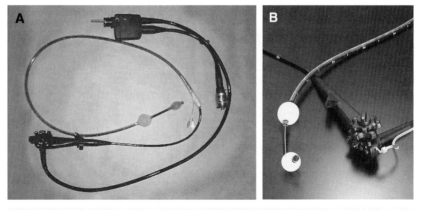

Fig. 3. (A) Double-balloon enteroscope. (B) Close-up view demonstrating latex balloons at the distal ends of the endoscope and overtube. (*Courtesy of* Fujinon, Inc.; with permission.)

The double balloon method is a system that warrants further explanation [17]. The overtube is backloaded onto the endoscope before intubation. Intubation of the endoscope is performed in the usual manner, with both balloons deflated. In the duodenum, the overtube balloon is inflated to hold the overtube in position. The endoscope then is advanced as far as possible. When the maximal depth of insertion is reached, the balloon on the tip of the endoscope is inflated. The overtube balloon then is deflated, and the overtube is advanced over the endoscope until its distal end approximates that of the endoscope. At this point, the overtube balloon is inflated, and the overtube and endoscope are gently pulled back. This causes pleating of the small intestine over the overtube/endoscope assembly and straightens the instrument. The endoscope balloon then is deflated; the endoscope is advanced further, and the entire process is repeated (Fig. 4). The goal is to reach the ileocecal valve, but this often is not achieved. If the entire small intestine is not intubated and it is clinically relevant, then a retrograde approach can be employed. Double balloon enteroscopy provides the opportunity for endoscopically directed therapy throughout the small intestine (Fig. 5). Double balloon enteroscopy from an oral approach requires no specific preparation other than a 6- to 8-hour fast before the procedure. If a retrograde approach is undertaken, a standard colon

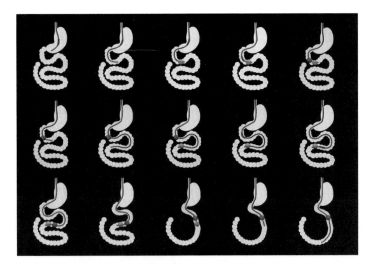

Fig. 4. Schematic demonstrating the steps in double-balloon enteroscopy. Intubation of the endoscope is performed with both balloons deflated. In the duodenum, the overtube balloon is inflated, and the endoscope is advanced. When the maximal depth of insertion is reached, the balloon on the tip of the endoscope is inflated. The overtube balloon then is deflated and the overtube advanced over the endoscope until its distal end approximates that of the endoscope. At this point, the overtube balloon is inflated, and both the overtube and the endoscope are pulled back gently, and the process is repeated. (*Courtesy of* Hironori Yamamoto, MD; and Fujinon, Inc.; with permission.)

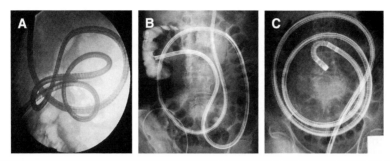

Fig. 5. (A) Fluoroscopic image taken during push enteroscopy compared with (B) double-balloon enteroscopy from an antegrade approach and (C) retrograde approach. Significantly less looping of the instrument occurs in double-balloon enteroscopy. (Photos 5B and 5C courtesy of Hironori Yamamoto, MD.)

preparation is necessary. Sedation may be achieved with standard conscious sedation, propofol, or general anesthesia.

Early reports by Yamamoto and colleagues using a prototype instrument [16,18] described results from 10 patients who had OGIB. Of eight patients who underwent double balloon enteroscopy using the 200 cm working length instrument, total enteroscopy (visualization of the entire small bowel) was achieved in three patients. In the other five patients, the procedure was terminated when it was felt that the diagnosis had been achieved. The source of bleeding was found in all patients, and no complications were reported. The investigators found the system to be easier to use with more comfortable handling than traditional enteroscopy. It was felt that the examination was less stressful to the patient, although this parameter was not evaluated formally. Like most technical procedures, there is a significant learning curve that affects the time needed to perform double balloon enteroscopy. A novice may require 2 to 3 hours, while an experienced practitioner may complete it in 75 to 90 minutes.

A larger series of 178 cases of double balloon enteroscopy in 123 patients was published by the same group in 2004 [19]. Fifty percent were performed in an antegrade fashion, and 50% were performed from a retrograde approach. GI bleeding was the indication for double balloon enteroscopy in 66 patients. Visualization of the entire small bowel was achieved in 86% of patients, and the source of bleeding was found in 76% of patients. Hemostasis using electrocautery was performed successfully in 12 cases. In the entire series of 178 procedures, two complications were reported (1.1%): multiple perforations in a patient who had intestinal lymphoma and prior chemotherapy, and post-procedure fever and abdominal pain in a patient who had Crohn's disease.

Multi-center experience with double balloon enteroscopy in the United States includes 47 procedures in 41 patients; 63% were done for the indication of GI bleeding. The mean procedure time was 115 minutes, and the mean distance obtained was 389 cm. The yield of double balloon enteroscopy for patients who had GI bleeding was 52%. Endoscopic hemostasis using argon beam photocoagulation or electrocautery was performed in five patients. In the entire series of 47 procedures, four complications were reported (8.5%): aspiration pneumonia, abdominal pain, unconfirmed microscopic perforation, and a jejunal tear (Jonathan Leighton, MD, unpublished data, 2005).

Intraoperative Enteroscopy

Intraoperative enteroscopy is the gold standard of small bowel imaging. The yield of detecting bleeding lesions in the small intestine reaches 83% to 100% [15], making it the most sensitive method of diagnosing small bowel disorders. The high sensitivity comes at the cost of extreme invasiveness, making it a procedure of last resort. Even at a major referral center, only about 10 intraoperative enteroscopy cases are performed each year for the indication of OGIB [20].

Intraoperative endoscopy is performed in conjunction with a surgeon in the operating room, with the patient under general anesthesia. An enteroscope or a pediatric colonoscope may be employed, depending on the anticipated route of intubation and the expected distance needed to traverse. Intubation may be achieved transorally, transanally, or through an operative enterotomy depending on clinical circumstance and physician preference. The endoscopist carefully inspects the intestinal lumen, while the surgeon examines the external wall with palpation and transillumination. Manipulation of the instrument is managed by the surgeon, who gently guides the intestine over the endoscope. Excellent communication and coordination between the surgeon and the gastroenterologist are required (Fig. 6). Examination of the mucosa is performed during the intubation, as trauma from the endoscope may mimic pathological lesions upon withdrawal. Minimizing air insufflation is important to keep the intestine pliable during the procedure and to limit traction on the mesentery. Lesions can be treated endoscopically or marked with a suture for surgical excision.

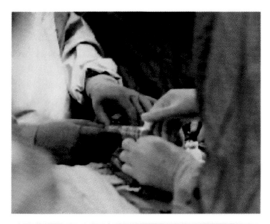

Fig. 6. Intraoperative enteroscopy. (*Courtesy of* Blair Lewis, MD.)

Complications of intraoperative enteroscopy include both those related to endoscopy and those related to major intestinal surgery. A review of 70 consecutive cases revealed an intraoperative complication rate of 3%, including one case of a mucosal tear and one case of intraoperative bleeding that was likely related to traction on the mesentery. In-hospital and 30-day mortality was 6%, with all deaths related to multi-system organ failure in the setting of ongoing bleeding. Postoperative complications occurred in 26% of patients, including prolonged ileus, transient atrial fibrillation, wound infection, myocardial infarction, respiratory failure, and deep vein thrombosis [20].

Before the advent of capsule endoscopy and double balloon endoscopy, intraoperative endoscopy was the only way to detect and treat lesions outside the reach of push enteroscopy. Now that less invasive techniques are available, the role of diagnostic intraoperative enteroscopy is likely to decrease, although it always will play a role in certain clinical scenarios.

Capsule Endoscopy

The difficulty encountered in attempts to navigate the small intestine with traditional flexible instruments led to the development of a new type of endoscope—one that could make its way through the 14 feet of small bowel without the restraint of a physical tether. Unbeknownst to each other, the idea of wireless imaging of the small intestine was conceived and pursued simultaneously by two independent researchers. Paul Swain, a British gastroenterologist, and Gavriel Iddan, an Israeli scientist, merged research efforts in 1998 and soon developed a pill-sized camera with sufficient battery life to image the entire small intestine [21]. Swain, in the tradition of many medical researchers, experimented on himself and was the first person to swallow a video capsule endoscope. The first patient trials were performed in April 2000, and their data were presented at the Digestive Disease Week in May of the same year. Capsule endoscopy became available commercially in the United States in August of 2001 and was an instant success.

The first commercially available video capsule is a part of the Given Diagnostic Imaging System (Given Imaging, Yoqneam, Israel). Other systems are being studied. The Given system is comprised of three main subsystems: an ingestible capsule endoscope, a data recorder, and a workstation. The PillCam SB (originally M2A) capsule measures 11 × 26 mm and weighs less than 4 g. This device captures two images per second and has a battery life of approximately 8 hours. After an overnight fast, the patient swallows the capsule, which travels through the GI tract by means of the actions of normal peristalsis. Images are transmitted by a digital radio frequency communication channel to an external data recorder unit.

The noninvasive nature of capsule endoscopy makes it an attractive option over traditional endoscopy. The examination requires little preparation, no sedation, causes no patient discomfort, and may provide a more physiologic view of the small intestine, because its movement is controlled by peristalsis. Furthermore, it has the ability to visualize the entirety of the small bowel mucosa, a feat otherwise limited to very invasive endoscopic procedures. The inherent disadvantage of capsule endoscopy is that it is a purely diagnostic test, with no capability for biopsy or therapeutic intervention. Patients can continue most of their usual activities during capsule endoscopy, making the test less disruptive than traditional endoscopy. Physician presence is not required during the exam, and the results may be interpreted at a convenient time.

The ideal preparation for capsule endoscopy continues to be a subject of debate. Ideal visualization of the mucosa may be marred by solid debris, liquid, bubbles, blood, or loss of battery life before reaching the cecum. The manufacturer recommends that patients start on a clear liquid diet after lunch the day before the procedure. Fasting is recommended for 8 hours before ingestion of the capsule, although pills may be taken with small sips of water.

Numerous agents have been used in an attempt to improve visualization of the mucosa during capsule endoscopy. A few small studies have used prokinetic agents or bowel preparation to mitigate these problems [22]. Oral sodium phosphate has been shown in a randomized series of 32 patients to decrease interference from intraluminal fluid [23]; however, there are concerns that it may increase gastric emptying time [24]. Simethicone given as a single 80 mg dose immediately before ingestion of the capsule improved visualization in one small randomized study [25]. Polyethylene glycol (PEG) increased visibility in the proximal small bowel in one study [26] but had no effect in another [27]. It may lead to more rapid transit through the stomach and small intestine [28]. Erythromycin leads to faster gastric emptying, but at the expense of slower small bowel transit time [29] and poorer visualization [24]. Tegaserod decreased small bowel transit time by 70 minutes in 18 patients [30]. Considerable variation exists in clinical practice, and the roles of bowel preparation and prokinetic agents will need to be addressed in larger studies.

The yield of capsule endoscopy in patients with OGIB ranges from 45% to 66% [14,31–35]. Determination of an accurate yield is hampered by the lack of a gold standard with which to compare capsule endoscopy. Most studies have compared capsule endoscopy with push enteroscopy, which is an imperfect comparison, because push enteroscopy is only capable of detecting lesions in the proximal small bowel. A more appropriate comparison would be with another procedure capable of examining the entire small intestine, such as intraoperative enteroscopy or double balloon enteroscopy. There is only one published report comparing capsule endoscopy with intraoperative enteroscopy. In 42 patients who had OGIB, intraoperative enteroscopy was performed within a week of capsule endoscopy. Sensitivity of both capsule endoscopy and intraoperative enteroscopy was 83%. There were no additional diagnoses made on intraoperative enteroscopy, although the authors described three patients in whom the extent of angiodysplasia was underestimated on capsule endoscopy [36] (Fig. 7).

There are nine published reports prospectively comparing the yield of capsule endoscopy with push enteroscopy [14,32,37–43]. The sensitivity of capsule endoscopy ranges from 55% to 76%, while the sensitivity of push enteroscopy

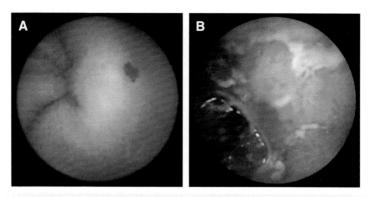

Fig. 7. Images from capsule endoscopy. (A) Angiodysplasia in the small intestine. (B) Small bowel ulceration and stricture.

ranges from 19% to 52%. A meta-analysis of 14 prospective trials comparing capsule endoscopy with push enteroscopy found an overall yield of 62% for capsule endoscopy versus 29% for push enteroscopy, with an incremental yield of 33% [34]. This relationship held for clinically significant findings, with the yield of capsule endoscopy 54% versus 24% for push enteroscopy, with an incremental yield of 30%. Capsule endoscopy has been reported to change patient management in up to 75% of cases [40].

Although capsule endoscopy is presumed to be tolerated better than traditional enteroscopy, there are few studies addressing this issue. In a questionnaire given to 21 patients undergoing both capsule endoscopy and push enteroscopy, none reported pain or discomfort, and all preferred capsule endoscopy over push enteroscopy [32]. Similarly, Mylonaki and colleagues found that 49 of 50 patients preferred capsule endoscopy to push enteroscopy, although two found the capsule uncomfortable to swallow [40]. Sixteen Asian patients rated the exam as comfortable and convenient [44].

The timing of capsule endoscopy in the patient who has OGIB has been addressed in two studies. When the capsule is administered to patients with ongoing overt bleeding, the yield is higher (87% to 92%) than in those with previous overt bleeding or iron deficiency anemia (46% to 56%) [33,45]. The high yield of capsule endoscopy, however, justifies this noninvasive test even if timing cannot be optimized.

The primary risk in capsule endoscopy is that of capsule entrapment within the GI tract (variously referred to as impaction and non-natural excretion). Entrapment occurs in 0.75% to 5% of cases [46,47]. Most capsule entrapment occurs in the small intestine, although case studies report impaction at the cricopharyngeus [48], tracheal aspiration [49,50], and retention in diverticulae [51,52]. Entrapment occurs nearly universally at the site of small bowel pathology, such that surgical intervention to retrieve the capsule also addresses the underlying problem. A trapped capsule may be retried endoscopically or may require surgical intervention. High-risk factors for entrapment include use of nonsteroidal anti-inflammatory drugs, prior abdominal radiation, Crohn's enteritis, and prior major abdominal surgery. Capsule entrapment in the small bowel is usually asymptomatic, even for several months [53], although disintegration of a retained capsule has been observed (David Fleischer, MD, personal communication, 2003).

The manufacturer lists the following contraindications to capsule endoscopy: patients with swallowing disorders, those with pacemakers or other implanted electromedical devices, and those with known or suspected gastrointestinal obstruction, stricture, or fistula. With new advances and more clinical experience, however, these difficulties are often surmountable. An endoscopic technique of capsule placement has been described for patients who are unable to swallow the capsule [54], and small series of capsule endoscopy in patients with pacemakers and implantable cardioverter defibrillators have failed to find harmful interaction between the devices [52,55,56]. Given Imaging is testing a patency system to try to prevent capsule entrapment in high-risk patients. The patency capsule is made of an ingestible, dissolvable capsule the same size as the Pill-Cam, and it contains a tiny radiofrequency identification tag. An external scanner can detect the presence and location of the patency capsule. Patients identified to be at risk for capsule entrapment will swallow the patency capsule, which will dissolve if it is unable to pass through the GI tract (Fig. 8).

To minimize the risk of capsule entrapment, a careful history should be taken, focusing on dysphagia or symptoms and risk factors for abdominal obstruction. A video esophagogram with administration of a 13 mm barium pill can detect those unlikely to successfully swallow the capsule. Until the patency system is commercially available, a barium small bowel series is recommended to rule out subclinical obstruction. Finally, in cases where the colon is not visualized on capsule endoscopy, and the patient does not see the capsule pass, an abdominal radiograph should be obtained to document passage of the capsule.

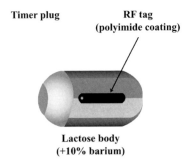

Fig. 8. Patency capsule. The radiofrequency tag allows for external detection of a retained capsule. The lactose body is designed to disintegrate within the GI tract within 2 to 3 days; barium within the body allows for radiographic detection.

OUTCOMES

A few small studies suggest that patient outcomes are improved after push enteroscopy. In 105 patients who had OGIB, resolution of bleeding occurred in 69% [57]. The mean follow-up was 29 months. Push enteroscopy influences the clinical management in 40% to 50% of patients who have OGIB [10,58]. Push enteroscopy with heater probe therapy of angiodysplasia has been shown to increase hemoglobin levels [59] and decrease transfusion requirements [60].

In 91 patients who had OGIB, capsule endoscopy led to treatment that resolved the bleeding in 87% [33]. The mean follow-up time was 18 months. Using the outcome measures of hospitalizations, blood transfusions, and procedures related to OGIB, a significant improvement was seen in patients who had occult and obscure GI bleeding after capsule endoscopy [45].

Resolution of GI bleeding occurred in 72% of patients in whom a lesion was found and treated on intraoperative enteroscopy [20]. Over a 32-month follow-up, bleeding persisted in 20% of patients and recurred in 8%. Eleven of 20 (55%) patients who underwent treatment of angiodysplasia on intraoperative enteroscopy were symptom-free at a mean of 11.6 months after the procedure [61]. These lesions are known to recur [62], however, making long-term outcome studies difficult to interpret in cases of OGIB caused by angiodysplasia.

DIRECTIONS FOR THE FUTURE

Numerous factors are being tested in an attempt to improve the diagnostic yield of capsule endoscopy. A longer battery life would reduce the number of incomplete studies. A capsule capable of capturing more images might yield more precise anatomic information. Other technologies such as real-time viewing and external control of the capsule could make capsule endoscopy an interactive process with active input from the gastroenterologist.

SUMMARY

The last frontier in luminal endoscopy has been conquered. Bleeding lesions in the small intestine can present a frustrating clinical problem, but recent advances have made investigating the small bowel easier and less invasive. Capsule endoscopy and double balloon enteroscopy are two new technologies that promise to lower the barrier to evaluation of the entire small intestine. Recent studies show that capsule endoscopy improves outcomes in patients who have OGIB. Although outcome studies regarding double balloon enteroscopy have not been performed, the opportunity to treat lesions throughout the small bowel without resorting to surgery is a tremendous advance. These improvements suggest that the corner may have been turned in the diagnosis and management of small bowel bleeding. Perhaps to the next generation of gastroenterologists, small bowel bleeding will not be obscure.

References

[1] Lewis BS. Small intestinal bleeding. Gastrointest Endosc Clin N Am 1994;23:67–91.

[2] Prakash C, Zuckerman GR. Acute small bowel bleeding: a distinct entity with significantly different economic implications compared with GI bleeding from other locations. Gastrointest Endosc 2003;58(3):330–5.

[3] Lewis BS. The history of enteroscopy. Gastrointest Endosc Clin N Am 1999;9(1):1–11.

[4] Seensalu R. The sonde exam. Gastrointest Endosc Clin N Am 1999;9:37–59.

[5] Taylor AC, Chen RY, Desmond PV. Use of an overtube for enteroscopy: does it increase depth of insertion? A prospective study of enteroscopy with and without an overtube. Endoscopy 2001;33:227–30.

[6] Harewood GC, Gostout CJ, Farrell MA, et al. Prospective controlled assessment of variable stiffness enteroscopy. Gastrointest Endosc 2003;58:267–71.

[7] Barkin JS, Lewis BS, Reiner DK, et al. Diagnostic and therapeutic jejunoscopy with a new, longer enteroscope. Gastrointest Endosc 1992;38:55–8.

[8] Keizman D, Brill S, Umansky M, et al. Diagnostic yield of routine push enteroscopy with a graded-stiffness enteroscope without overtube. Gastrointest Endosc 2003;57:877–81.

[9] Berner JS, Mauer K, Lewis BS. Push and sonde enteroscopy for the diagnosis of obscure gastrointestinal bleeding. Am J Gastroenterol 1994;89(12):2139–42.

[10] Bezet A, Cuillerier E, Landi B, et al. Clinical impact of push enteroscopy in patients with gastrointestinal bleeding of unknown origin. Clin Gastroenterol Hepatol 2004;2(10):921–7.

[11] Taylor AC, Buttigieg RJ, McDonald IG, et al. Prospective assessment of the diagnostic and therapeutic impact of small-bowel push enteroscopy. Endoscopy 2003;35(11):951–6.

[12] Perry SD, Welfare MR, Cobden I, et al. Push enteroscopy in a UK district general hospital: experience of 51 cases over 2 years. Eur J Gastroenterol Hepatol 2002;14:305–9.

[13] Landi B, Tkoub M, Gaudric M, et al. Diagnostic yield of push-type enteroscopy in relation to indication. Gut 1998;42:421–5.

[14] Ell C, Remke S, May A, et al. The first prospective controlled trial comparing wireless capsule endoscopy with push enteroscopy in chronic gastrointestinal bleeding. Endoscopy 2002;34(9):685–9.

[15] Swain P, Fritscher-Ravens A. Role of video endoscopy in managing small bowel disease. Gut 2004;53:1866–75.

[16] Yamamoto H, Sekine Y, Sato Y, et al. Total enteroscopy with a nonsurgical steerable double-balloon method. Gastrointest Endosc 2001;53(2):216–20.

[17] Yamamoto H, Sugano K. A new method of enteroscopy-The double-balloon method. Can J Gastroenterol 2003;17(4):273–4.

[18] May A, Nachbar L, Wardak A, et al. Double balloon enteroscopy: preliminary experience in patients with obscure gastrointestinal bleeding or chronic abdominal pain. Endoscopy 2003;35(12):985–91.

[19] Yamamoto H, Kita H, Sunada K, et al. Clinical outcomes of double balloon endoscopy for the diagnosis and treatment of small intestinal diseases. Clin Gastroenterol Hepatol 2004;2:1010–6.

[20] Kendrick ML, Buttar NS, Anderson MA, et al. Contribution of intraoperative enteroscopy in the management of obscure gastrointestinal bleeding. J Gastrointest Surg 2001;5(2):162–7.

[21] Iddan GJ, Swain CP. History and development of capsule endoscopy. Gastrointest Endosc Clin N Am 2004;14(1):1–9.

[22] Rosch T. DDW Report 2004 New Orleans: capsule endoscopy. Endoscopy 2004;36(9):763–9.

[23] Niv Y, Abuksis G. Capsule endoscopy: role of bowel preparation in successful visualization. [abstract]. Gastroenterology 2004;126:A-461.

[24] Fireman Z, Paz D. Capsule endoscopy: improving the transit time and the image view [abstract]. Gastrointest Endosc 2004;59(5):AB173.

[25] Albert J, Gobel CM, Lesske J, et al. Simethicone for small bowel preparation for capsule endoscopy: a systematic, single-blinded, controlled study. Gastrointest Endosc 2004; 59:487.

[26] Chong A, Miller A, Taylor A, et al. Randomised controlled trial of polyethyelene glycol administration prior to capsule endoscopy [abstract]. Gastrointest Endosc 2004;59(5):AB179.

[27] Soussan EB, Antonietti M, Lecleire S, et al. Influence of bowel preparation for capsule endoscopy: quality of examination and transit time [abstract]. Gastrointest Endosc 2004; 59(5):AB178.

[28] Fireman Z, Kopelman Y, Fish L, et al. Effect of oral purgatives on gastric and small bowel transit time in capsule endoscopy. Isr Med Assoc J 2004;6:521–3.

[29] Coumaros D, Claudel L, Levy P, et al. Diagnostic value of capsule endoscopy (CE) in obscure digestive bleeding (ODB) and effect of erythromycin injection [abstract]. Gastrointest Endosc 2004;59(5):AB177.

[30] Schmelkin IJ. Tegaserod decreases small bowel transit times in patients undergoing capsule endoscopy [abstract]. Gastrointest Endosc 2004;59(5):AB176.

[31] Costamagna G, Shah SK, Riccioni ME, et al. A prospective trial comparing small bowel radiographs and video capsule endoscopy for suspected small bowel disease. Gastroenterology 2002;123:999–1005.

[32] Lewis BS, Swain P. Capsule endoscopy in the evaluation of patients with suspected small intestinal bleeding: results of a pilot study. Gastrointest Endosc 2002;56(3):349–53.

[33] Pennazio M, Santucci R, Rondonotti E, et al. Outcome of patients with obscure gastrointestinal bleeding after capsule endoscopy: report of 100 consecutive patients. Gastroenterology 2004;126:643–53.

[34] Triester SL, Leighton JA, Fleischer DE, et al. Yield of capsule endoscopy compared to other modalities in patients with obscure GI bleeding: a meta-analysis. Am J Gastroenterol 2004;99:A941.

[35] Enns R, Go K, Chang H, et al. Capsule endoscopy: a single centre experience with the first 226 capsules. Can J Gastroenterol 2004;18(9):555–8.

[36] Bolz G, Schmitt H, Hartmann D, et al. Prospective controlled trial comparing wireless capsule endoscopy with intraoperative enteroscopy in patients with chronic gastrointestinal bleeding: ongoing multicenter study. Presented at the 3rd International Conference on Capsule Endoscopy, Miami, FL, March 1, 2004.

[37] Saurin JC, Delvaux M, Gaudin JL, et al. Diagnostic value of endoscopic capsule in patients with obscure digestive bleeding: blinded comparison with video push enteroscopy. Endoscopy 2003;35:576–84.

[38] Adler DG, Knipschield M, Gostout C. A prospective comparison of capsule endoscopy and push enteroscopy in patients with GI bleeding of obscure origin. Gastrointest Endosc 2004;59(4):492–8.

[39] Van Gossum A, Hittelet A, Schmit A, et al. A prospective comparative study of push and wireless-capsule enteroscopy in patients with obscure digestive bleeding. Acta Gastroenterol Belg 2003;66(3):199–205.

[40] Mylonaki M, Fritscher-Ravens A, Swain P. Wireless capsule endoscopy: a comparison with push enteroscopy in patients with gastroscopy and colonoscopy negative gastrointestinal bleeding. Gut 2003;52:1122–6.

[41] Hartmann D, Schilling D, Bolz G, et al. Capsule endoscopy versus push enteroscopy in patients with occult gastrointestinal bleeding. Z Gastroenterol 2003;41(5):377–82.

[42] Mata A, Bordas JM, Few F, et al. Wireless capsule endoscopy in patients with obscure gastrointestinal bleeding: a comparative study with push enteroscopy. Aliment Pharmacol Ther 2004;20:189–94.

[43] Ge ZZ, Hu YB, Xiao SD. Capsule endoscopy and push enteroscopy in the diagnosis of obscure gastrointestinal bleeding. Chin Med J (Engl) 2004;117(7):1045–9.

[44] Ang TL, Fock KM, Ng TM, et al. Clinical utility, safety and tolerability of capsule endoscopy in urban Southeast Asian population. World J Gastroenterol 2003;9(10):2313.

[45] Carey EJ, Leighton JA, Heigh RI, et al. Single center outcomes of 260 consecutive patients undergoing capsule endoscopy for obscure GI bleeding. Gastroenterology 2004;126(4): A96.

[46] Barkin JS, Friedman S. Wireless capsule requiring surgical intervention. The world's experience. Am J Gastroenterol 2002;97(9):A83.

[47] Pennazio M. Small-bowel Endoscopy. Endoscopy 2004;36(1):32–41.

[48] Fleischer DE, Heigh RI, Nguyen CC, et al. Video capsule impaction at the cricopharyngeus: a first report of this complication and its successful resolution. Gastrointest Endosc 2003;57(3):427–8.

[49] Tabib S, Fuller C, Daniels J, et al. Asymptomatic aspiration of a capsule endoscope. Gastrointest Endosc 2004;60(5):845–8.

[50] Sinn I, Neef B, Andus T. Aspiration of a capsule endoscope. Gastrointest Endosc 2004;59(7):926–7.

[51] Feitoza AB, Gostout CJ, Knipschield MA, et al. Video capsule endoscopy—is the recording time ideal? Am J Gastroenterol 2002;97(Suppl 1):S307.

[52] Barkin JS, O'Loughlin C. Capsule endoscopy contraindications: complications and how to avoid their occurrence. Gastrointest Endosc Clin N Am 2004;14(1):61–5.

[53] Taylor A, Miller A, Woods R, et al. Long-term retained capsule without ill effects in a patient with ileal ulceration and undiagnosed stricture. In: Jacob H, editor. Proceedings of the first Given Conference, Rome 2002. Haifa (Israel): Rochash Printing; 2003. p. 115.

[54] Carey EJ, Heigh RI, Fleischer DE. Endoscopic capsule endoscope delivery for patients with dysphagia, anatomical abnormalities, or gastroparesis. Gastrointest Endosc 2004;59(3): 423–6.

[55] Leighton JA, Srivathsan K, Carey EJ, et al. Safety of wireless capsule endoscopy in patients with implantable cardiac defibrillators. Am J Gastroenterol 2005;100:1728–31.

[56] Leighton JA, Sharma VK, Srivathsan K, et al. Safety of capsule endoscopy in patients with pacemakers. Gastrointest Endosc 2004;59(4):567–9.

[57] Landi B, Cellier C, Gaudric M, et al. Long-term outcome of patients with gastrointestinal bleeding of obscure origin explored by push enteroscopy. Endoscopy 2001;34(5):355–9.

[58] Hayat M, Axon AT, O'Mahony S. Diagnostic yield and effect on clinical outcomes of push enteroscopy in suspected small-bowel bleeding. Endoscopy 2000;32(5):369–72.

[59] Morris AJ, Mokhashi M, Straiton M, et al. Push enteroscopy and heater probe therapy for small bowel bleeding. Gastrointest Endosc 1996;44:394–7.

[60] Vakil N, Huilgol V, Khan I. Effect of push enteroscopy on transfusion requirements and quality of life in patients with unexplained gastrointestinal bleeding. Am J Gastroenterol 1997;92(3):425–8.

[61] Lewis BS, Wenger JS, Waye JD. Small bowel enteroscopy and intraoperative enteroscopy for obscure gastrointestinal bleeding. Am J Gastroenterol 1991;86(2):171–4.

[62] Zuckerman GR, Prakash C, Askin MP, et al. Technical review: the evaluation and management of occult and obscure GI bleeding. Gastroenterology 2000;118:201–21.

ELSEVIER
SAUNDERS

Gastroenterol Clin N Am 34 (2005) 735–752

GASTROENTEROLOGY CLINICS
OF NORTH AMERICA

Angiographic Diagnosis and Endovascular Management of Nonvariceal Gastrointestinal Hemorrhage

Michael Miller, Jr, MD*, Tony P. Smith, MD

Department of Radiology, Duke University Medical Center, Room 1502, Box 3808, Durham, NC 27710, USA

The diagnostic angiographic approach to acute nonvariceal gastrointestinal (GI) hemorrhage is philosophically different for the upper versus the lower GI tracts. Angiography has a small role in the diagnosis of upper GI bleeding, limited to those situations where endoscopy cannot localize a bleeding site. Such endoscopic failure for the esophagus, stomach, and duodenum are most often related to anatomical situations preventing full endoscopy, such as impassable strictures and surgical alterations of anatomy. Angiography plays a larger diagnostic role for patients with lower GI bleeding when endoscopy and other imaging modalities are not able to satisfactorily locate the site and etiology of bleeding. Most important, diagnostic angiography today is most often a precursor to transcatheter therapy, which has become an important weapon in the armamentarium for the treatment of acute GI bleeding. This review focuses on the current roles of diagnostic angiography and transcatheter therapy for the patient with nonvariceal GI bleeding.

ANATOMY AND ANGIOGRAPHIC DIAGNOSIS

Angiography for GI bleeding using percutaneous catheterization techniques was first performed in patients by Baum and colleagues in 1965, identifying hemorrhage as contrast extravasation into the bowel in four of their eight patients [1]. Although the techniques, tools, and radiographic equipment have changed significantly since that time, the angiographic diagnosis is still based on the same perception of contrast material collecting in the lumen of the bowel.

This review focuses on the current roles of diagnostic angiography and transcatheter therapy for the patient with nonvariceal gastrointestinal bleeding.

*Corresponding author. E-mail address: mille052@mc.duke.edu (M. Miller).

0889-8553/05/$ – see front matter
doi:10.1016/j.gtc.2005.09.001

Angiography remains the radiographic gold standard for the diagnosis of GI bleeding, and its specificity approaches 100%. It provides imaging of the entire mesenteric system, localizes the site or sites of hemorrhage, and affords the opportunity for transcatheter therapy. In addition, angiography allows visualization of other rarer sites of hemorrhage, such as the biliary tree [2]. However, there are many problems with angiography for the diagnosis of upper and lower GI bleeding. First, it is an invasive procedure that is uncomfortable for the patient and has a finite complication rate. Complications include those associated with any angiographic procedure, such as access site thrombosis or hemorrhage, contrast reactions, and injury to the target vessels, specifically the superior mesenteric artery (SMA), inferior mesenteric artery (IMA), and celiac artery including dissection and distal embolization. The overall rate of complication for mesenteric angiography is similar to most selective angiography and is acceptable at less than 5%, including access site complications and arterial dissections [3]. In addition, one could assume these figures are now somewhat dated given advances in guide wire and catheter technology. However, Cohn and colleagues found that of 65 patients undergoing 75 selective angiograms for evaluation of acute lower GI bleeding, angiography-related complications occurred in seven patients (11%), but this included findings such as on-table abdominal pain and incisional hemorrhage secondary to urokinase and heparin administration while attempting to induce bleeding [4].

Diagnostic angiography for upper GI bleeding is straightforward and centers on the anatomy of the celiac artery. Specifically, the celiac gives rise to the left gastric artery, which provides branches to the distal esophagus and fundus of the stomach (Fig. 1). These branches also communicate with distal branches of the small short gastric arteries from the splenic artery and branches of the right gastric artery. The latter is usually a small artery that originates from the left or common hepatic artery but is often not visualized angiographically. The remainder of the stomach and duodenum are supplied by branches from the gastroduodenal artery. The SMA may supply portions of the duodenum mostly via pancreaticoduodenal anatomoses, which for the most part are important angiographically as a rich collateral supply keeping the stomach and duodenum viable following celiac branch embolization, but also may be responsible for rehemorrhage following embolotherapy. Anatomical variations in the celiac anatomy occur in at least 50% of the population, most notably in the origins of the hepatic arteries (see Fig. 1). Such variations must always be considered when evaluating a patient angiographically for GI bleeding.

In the setting of upper GI bleeding, the source for hemorrhage is usually identified by endoscopy. Therefore, angiography is most often performed only as a precursor to transcatheter embolotherapy based on the known vascular supply to the area of abnormality. As with angiography in the lower GI tract, a positive examination is classically described as extravasation of contrast into the bowel lumen. However, an abnormal blush of the mucosal surface of the upper GI tract is indicative of an inflammatory process (gastritis or duodenitis), which, if correlated with endoscopy findings, may also be considered

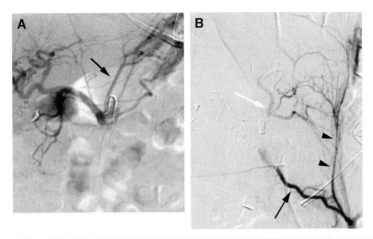

Fig. 1. Two separate patients with upper gastrointestinal bleeding. (A) Patient with upper GI bleeding and normal-appearing left gastric artery (*arrow*). (B) A 75-year-old man with recurrent bleeding post-Whipple procedure and prior embolization of the gastroduodenal and common hepatic arteries who on left gastric injection demonstrates collateral (*arrowheads*) filling of the hepatic artery (*white arrow*) from the left gastric artery (*black arrow*).

a positive angiographic examination. Angiography in the setting of upper GI bleeding is positive for extravasation or abnormal mucosal blush in up to 61% of cases [5,6]. This limited sensitivity for acute bleeding is not problematic, as it is generally believed that empiric embolization of a targeted vascular bed is safe and effective, thus decreasing the prerequisite for positive angiography.

Diagnostic angiography for lower GI bleeding centers on the anatomy of the superior and inferior mesenteric vessels that supply the bowel distal to the ligament of Treitz, with the watershed area between the two usually in the left one-third of the transverse colon. The IMA subsequently supplies the descending and sigmoid colon to the rectum, which has a variable supply from numerous sources. In general, extravasation indicative of a hemorrhage occurs in about 50% of patients presenting with acute lower GI hemorrhage, although reports of vascular abnormalities suggestive of a bleeding site have been found in an additional 32% of patients [7,8]. Low sensitivity for diagnostic angiography is a much greater issue in the patient with lower GI bleeding and is a multifaceted problem. Following the diagnosis of acute GI bleeding based on clinical, endoscopic, and imaging findings, it is usually a prolonged interval until the patient undergoes an angiographic study. During usual working hours, the angiographic suites may already have patients, resulting in a variable delay. During off-hours, in most medical centers a call team needs to be mobilized. Given the intermittent nature of bleeding, the likelihood of finding a bleeding site often decreases. Finally, angiography can diagnose a bleeding site only when there is a rapid rate of bleeding. This is understandable in that the contrast material is only in the arterial system for a few seconds and there must be enough extravasation into the bowel to be seen radiographically. That bleeding rate must be at least 1 mL/min, although that number is controversial; it is said to be too low by some and too high by others [9]. Regardless, it is clear to all that a substantial amount of bleeding at the precise time of contrast injection is required before an angiographic diagnosis can be achieved.

Angiography for GI bleeding is usually performed from a common femoral artery access. Upper extremity arterial access can be used when femoral access is not possible, and may even be necessary as it often provides better angles for catheterization of mesenteric vessels relative to the abdominal aorta. Angiography for GI bleeding is most often performed with 5 French catheter systems of which there are various useful shapes. Aortography is seldom necessary unless there is difficulty with selective catheterization. Selective catheterization for upper GI bleeding includes the celiac and superior mesenteric arteries, whereas lower GI bleeding includes the superior and inferior mesenteric arteries. The initial artery catheterized is the one most suspected of bleeding based on prior imaging or endoscopy, which is of course the celiac for upper GI bleeding. For lower GI bleeding, if bleeding from the descending and sigmoid colon is suspected, then inferior mesenteric angiography should be performed initially. Certainly, if a bleeding site is not found in the primary areas of suspicion, the remaining bowel distribution should be evaluated angiographically such that all three vessels supplying the mesentery have been thoroughly studied. In the authors' practice, even if a bleeding site is located in a single vessel distribution, angiography of all three vessels is performed to exclude a second site and to thoroughly understand the anatomy, including diseased segments and potential for collateral supply to the bleeding site and possible embolotherapy. For the patient with lower GI bleeding, if a bleeding site is not found in the acute setting, the patient may return to the care unit with an arterial access sheath in place to facilitate a second study should bleeding recur. Access to the common femoral artery may also be left in place up to 24 hours even in light of a successful embolization in the setting of coagulopathy or a high concern for recurrent life-threatening hemorrhage.

There is much discussion about the necessity of diagnostic studies preceding angiography. Certainly, endoscopy has a diagnostic and therapeutic role and can completely replace the need for angiography of the upper GI tract in greater than 90% of patients [10]. However, most of the controversy involves the need for nuclear scintigraphy before diagnostic angiography in the patient with lower GI bleeding. Scinitgraphy has been notoriously inaccurate when locating lesions for surgical resection; however, scintigraphy is certainly more sensitive, requiring reportedly 10-fold less hemorrhage than angiography to achieve a positive study [11]. As an adjunct to angiography, the probability of a positive diagnostic angiogram is increased by a preceding positive nuclear scintigraphic study. Gunderman and colleagues, in a retrospective review, found scintigraphic screening appeared to increase by a factor of 2.4 the diagnostic yield of arteriography by screening out patients who are not actively bleeding at the time of the examination, thus sparing them the risks and costs of a nondiagnostic invasive study [12]. There also appears to be a correlation linking positive angiography to a shortened interval between injection of the radiotracer and the identification of tracer activity signifying a bleed. Unfortunately, this has not been confirmed by controlled patient series at this time. In general, the decision to proceed directly to angiography without nuclear scintigraphy depends on the clinical situation and the degree of hemorrhage. The clinical presentation of lower GI bleeding may be episodic or continual. The former ranges from minor episodes that resolve, to chronic intermittent bleeding, to severe life-threatening hemorrhage. Angiography is warranted in the latter group and may, with provocation, play a diagnostic role in the second. In the authors' center, nuclear scintigraphy is recommended before angiography in all cases of episodic bleeding. Angiography remains the primary diagnostic imaging tool in those patients with continual active hemorrhage, however, and delaying angiography for scintigraphy is not warranted.

Intermittent lower gastrointestinal hemorrhage deserves special attention. This difficult group of patients often bleeds, frequently to low hemoglobin and hematocit levels, yet a site cannot be localized. Bleeding has been successfully provoked using a variable combination of anticoagulants, vasodilators, and fibrinolytics [13]. The authors' center has reported 16 such patients with occult lower GI bleeding, and bleeding was provoked in six (38%) without complication [14]. Such early data clearly requires further study but does represent a promising diagnostic approach to patients with an extremely difficult clinical problem.

TRANSCATHETER INTERVENTION: UPPER GASTROINTESTINAL HEMORRHAGE

Transcatheter intervention to control GI bleeding takes two forms: the infusion of a vasoconstricting medication and the mechanical occlusion of the arterial supply responsible for the hemorrhage. Vasopressin, a posterior pituitary hormone, elicits smooth muscle contraction in the mesenteric bed, thereby decreasing the perfusion pressure to the bowel and potentially resulting in thrombosis of the bleeding site. Vasopressin infusion is easy to perform, most often by placing a 5 F diagnostic catheter into the artery most suspected of bleeding, traditionally the left gastric although placement in the celiac artery is acceptable given the extremely low rates of hepatic and splenic organ ischemia [15]. The infusion technique is then identical to that for lower GI bleeding. Vasopressin infusion has lost favor for two main reasons: necessary catheterization times can require several days and, more importantly, the emergence of embolotherapy. For nonvariceal upper GI bleeding, the offending arteries—namely, the left gastric and gastroduodenal—were easily accessible even with, by today's standards, large and crude catheter systems and embolic agents. In addition, given the rich arterial collateral network and proximal site of embolotherapy, ischemia was not thought to be problematic.

Given that embolotherapy replaced vasopressin infusion early in the treatment of upper GI bleeding, there is little recent data on the use of this agent.

In addition, much of the data combines the treatment of variceal bleeding. A review of four of the more recent studies from 1979 to 1984 consisting of 267 patients demonstrated an initial 70% to 80% success rate with an approximate 20% rate of rehemorrhage with bleeding refractory to infusion in up to 40% of patients [16–19]. Eckstein and colleagues infused the left gastric artery in 155 patients and the celiac in 20 with a success rate of 75% for the left gastric and 80% for the celiac, with rehemorrhage in 18% and 19%, respectively [19]. Complications occurred in 6.5%, mostly related to arterial access but notably no cases of bowel ischemia. Sherman and colleagues, using vasopressin infusion, had initial treatment success in 12 of 15 patients with gastritis (80%), 6 of 11 with ulcer disease (55%), and 0 of 1 with Mallory-Weiss tear (0%) [16]. Complete control occurred in 66%, 46%, and 0%, respectively, finding the best results in the gastritis group. Their major complication rate was 34%, consisting mostly of pulmonary edema and myocardial depression without bowel ischemia. Clark and colleagues reported 43 patients infused with vasopressin for upper GI hemorrhage, and 32 (74%) were controlled, although with supplemental embolotherapy in three [17]. The authors concluded primary vasopressin with embolization for failures or contraindications is more effective than either therapy alone. Failures of vasopressin are thought to be due to the rich collateral supply to the upper GI tract and the inability to treat potential collateral supply pathways to the bleeding site, but this is unproven. The recurrence rate in these studies is not so dissimilar to those of transcatheter embolotherapy.

Studies that directly compare the results of vasopressin therapy are scarce and possess small patient numbers. Dahl and colleagues randomized 30 patients, 15 with mucosal lesions to intravenous vasopressin (n = 10) versus no therapy (n = 5) [18]. The remaining 15 had variceal bleeding. They found bleeding subsided in 7 of 10 patients receiving vasopressin but in 0 of 5 controls, prompting the authors to conclude that vasopressin was useful in controlling mucosal hemorrhage [18]. Another study attempted to compare patients retrospectively in a single center using intraarterial transcatheter techniques as described here. Gomes and colleagues retrospectively compared 14 patients receiving vasopressin for stomach or duodenal bleeding to 11 patients receiving embolization [20]. Primary success occurred in 10 patients (71%) with vasopressin versus 7 (64%) with embolotherapy, whereas only one complication occurred in each group. However, rebleeding occurred in four (40%) patients treated with vasopressin compared with only one (14%) undergoing embolotherapy, prompting the authors to conclude that embolization should be used as the primary method for angiographic control of the bleeding vessel when it could be selectively catheterized. Stump and Hardin in their 1990 review of the use of vasopressin in the treatment of upper gastrointestinal hemorrhage concluded that the use of vasopressin in nonvariceal upper GI bleeding would be empiric as there is no substantial data to support its use [21]. In the authors' opinion, no studies of substance have been published since that time to change this viewpoint.

The first transcatheter embolization for upper GI bleeding was of the right gastroepiploic artery using autologous clot reported by Rösch and colleagues in 1972 [22]. Embolization for upper GI bleeding could be performed via large diagnostic angiography catheters with proximal agents, and many of these same techniques are used today. Proximal embolic agents can be divided into two main groups: temporary and permanent. Temporary agents are those that are absorbed by the body and are touted to be ideal agents for patients with upper GI bleeding because the underlying problem, such as peptic ulcer disease, can be eventually cured. Thus if one uses a temporary agent, the artery recannalizes itself and in effect preserves an intact arterial supply to the stomach or duodenum. Chief among the temporary agents are gelatin sponge (Gelfoam; Pharmacia & Upjohn Co., Kalamazoo, Michigan) and autologous clot. Both agents require large bore diagnostic catheters, which can be difficult to place in some patients, and the administration of these agents is not precise. More permanent agents, such as coils, are radiopaque and allow better control of placement. In addition, new microcatheter systems, as discussed for lower GI bleeding, allow catheterization of small and tortuous systems and permit more precise placement of microcoils or even the injection of various particulates, such as polyvinyl alcohol sponge or gelatin spheres. However, there has been little published on the efficacy of the different embolic materials in head-to-head comparisons. In the setting of coagulopathy there is some data to suggest that the combination of particles and coils may be more effective in achieving clinical success than coils alone [5].

Regardless of the technical aspects of the procedure, transcatheter embolotherapy has become the mainstay for the radiographic treatment of nonvariceal upper GI bleeding, and is second only to endoscopic measures in most centers (Fig. 2). Although much of the information regarding the success of embolotherapy is dated, nine publications since 1990, consisting of 434 patients, have been reviewed in an attempt to ascertain more recent figures (see Refs. [5,6,23–29]). Unfortunately, because of the differences in study design and reporting, a full comprehensive analysis is not reliably obtainable. But some useful information can be gleamed from these reports. In general, technical success for embolotherapy was greater than 95% when reported, and clinical success ranged from 52% to 91% depending on the individual study's definitions. In the largest series, Schenker and colleagues reported on 163 patients and achieved target vessel devascularization in 155 (95%) and clinical success in 95 (58%) [6]. Some reports have suggested greater success in one arterial distribution versus another. Lang reported on 13 patients over a 5-year period with massive upper GI hemorrhage and a normal angiogram [24]. Seven patients underwent embolization; two of these rehemorrhaged, and six had conservative therapy, resulting in rebleeding in four [7]. When the left gastric artery was the target vessel, rehemorrhage did not occur following embolization (n = 6) versus two of four receiving conservative treatment. Alternatively, Toyoda and colleagues reported on 11 patients who had duodenal hemorrhage refractory to endoscopic therapy and underwent embolization of the gastroduodenal

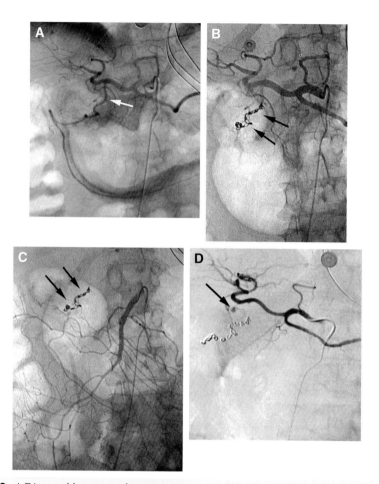

Fig. 2. A 76-year-old woman with upper gastrointestinal bleeding and hemodynamic instability despite endoscopic intervention for a duodenal ulcer. (A) Diagnostic arteriogram of the celiac artery was without extravasation from the gastroduodenal artery (GDA) (arrow). (B) Celiac arteriogram following empiric coil embolization (arrows) of the gastroduodenal artery. (C) Superior mesenteric arteriogram confirming absent collateral filling of the GDA (arrows). (D) Four days later, the patient presents with recurrent bleeding. Celiac arteriogram demonstrating extravasation of contrast (arrow). (E) Microcatheter (arrowheads) selection of the source vessel with extravasation (arrow). (F) Branch coil embolization (arrow) through the microcatheter (arrowheads). (G) Celiac arteriogram confirming occlusion of the source vessel (arrow).

artery [27]. Ten of 11 patients (91%) were controlled; the other could only receive proximal gastroduodenal occlusion because of atherosclerosis and rehemorrhaged distal to the embolization from collaterals [10]. No ischemic complications were noted on follow-up endoscopy performed on all patients. Walsh and colleagues reported a total of 47 patients who were embolized for

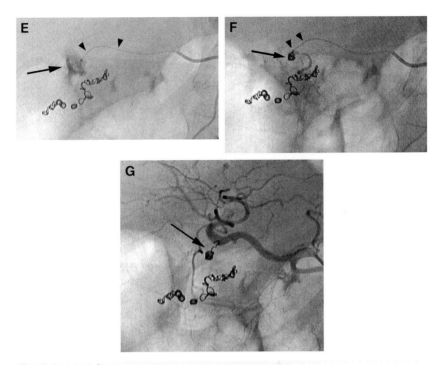

Fig. 2 (continued)

massive gastroduodenal hemorrhage and found no difference regarding the source (stomach versus duodenum) or whether active bleeding was found at angiography [28].

Although not as worrisome as with lower gastrointestinal embolotherapy, ischemia does occur in the upper GI tract following embolization. Aina and colleagues reviewed 75 consecutive patients who underwent arterial embolization for upper GI bleeding and reported a 99% technical success with a primary clinical success in 76% [5]. However, three cases (4%) of ischemia were noted, two involving the duodenum and one the liver. Encarnacion and colleagues retrospectively reviewed 36 embolization procedures in 29 patients; 25 of these were the left gastric [14] or gastroduodenal [11] arteries, the remainder in the superior mesenteric [26]. A single patient had endoscopic evidence of duodenal ischemia following gastroduodenal embolization but remained asymptomatic. Lang reported control of duodenal hemorrhage using a multitude of agents, including liquid, particulate, and coils in 52 of 57 patients [25]. Distal agents, including glue, were successful in controlling hemorrhage in 15 of 28 (54%) versus 8 of 29 (28%) using proximal agents. However, the distal agents resulted in duodenal stenoses from ischemia in 7 of 28 (25%) versus 2 of 29 (7%) for the more proximal arterial occlusions. Lieberman and colleagues retrospectively reviewed their series of 32 patients embolized for upper GI bleeding, 27 (84%) of whom had active bleeding by diagnostic angiography. Twenty-three patients (72%), four without active bleeding and 19 with active bleeding, were initially controlled by embolotherapy [30]. Eight patients with active bleeding and one without could not be controlled. Of those successfully embolized, four rehemorrhaged within 24 hours. Two patients had gastric necrosis and one had new gastric ulcerations, all indicative of ischemia. All three had surgically altered anatomy and were embolized with gelatin sponge powder, which is a distal agent of variable particle size.

Unlike lower GI tract bleeding, the need for angiographic confirmation of a bleeding site is not a prerequisite for transcatheter therapy in the upper GI tract (see Fig. 2). Two studies looking at the factors determining clinical success of embolotherapy for the treatment of upper GI bleeding showed no difference between empiric embolization based on surgical or endoscopic guidance without extravasation and those patients with positive angiography [5,6], although an earlier third study did not agree [23]. All three studies did, however, find positive impact on survival when embolization was successful in the setting of extravasation of contrast, confirming the current practice of almost all centers to empirically embolize the most likely offending vessel based on endoscopic guidance (see Fig. 2).

Predictors of clinical failure to control upper GI bleeding seem to agree that coagulopathy and multiorgan failure result in a reduced likelihood of clinical success. Schenker and colleagues found a 17.5-fold mortality rate in patients with multiorgan failure and upper GI bleeding [6]. However, patients with multiorgan failure and successful embolization had a 69% rate of survival compared with a 4% rate of survival when embolization failed, prompting the authors to conclude that embolization should be attempted in these patients despite their higher mortality rate. Coagulopathy has been shown to adversely impact the success rate for embolotherapy with an increase in odds ratio for clinical failure, which ranges from 2.9 to 19.6 [5,6,26]. However, aggressive correction of coagulation factors before embolization and distal vascular occlusion with particles may improve efficacy in patients with such disorders [5].

Many of the reporting difficulties relate to the lack of studies that have prospectively compared transcatheter therapy with other treatment modalities. Ripoll and colleagues recently attempted to retrospectively compare transcatheter embolotherapy for the treatment of upper GI bleeding refractory to endoscopic intervention with surgery [29]. Although there was no difference in the rate of recurrent bleeding (20% versus 23%), the need for additional surgery (16% versus 30.8%), or death (25.8% versus 20.5%) between the two, the embolotherapy group was treating significantly older patients ($P < 0.001$) with more comorbidities, such as heart disease ($P < 0.001$) and prior anticoagulation therapy ($P = .018$). There is clearly a great need for prospective studies in the endovascular management of bleeding from the upper GI tract.

TRANSCATHETER INTERVENTION: LOWER GASTROINTESTINAL HEMORRHAGE

Not long after angiography was being routinely performed for the diagnosis of lower GI bleeding, attempts were made at transcatheter control of the hemorrhage. As with upper GI bleeding, two techniques have been used: the infusion of a vasoconstricting agent (vasopressin) and transcatheter embolotherapy. Baum and colleagues described the technique of using vasopressin to control lower gastrointestinal bleeding in 1972 [31]. There are few contraindications to vasopressin infusion—the main one based in large part on constriction of other diseased arterial beds, most notably the coronary circulation. Vasopressin infusion has the advantage of being technically easy to perform. A 5 French diagnostic catheter is simply placed in the proximal SMA or IMA and infusion is begun. The rate of infusion is somewhat center specific but also varies according to an individual patient's angiographic vasoconstrictive response (Fig. 3). In general, infusion typically begins with 0.1 to 0.2 units/min and is increased from that point [9]. Patients are kept on the angiographic table for 20-minute infusion intervals, after which angiography is performed to assess the level of vasoconstriction and the response of the bleeding site (see Fig. 3). Severe vasoconstriction necessitates a lower dose, continued bleeding a larger dose—typically not to exceed 0.4 units/min. Once a reasonable vasoconstrictive effect is achieved, patients are transferred to an intensive care unit where infusion is continued for 12 hours, at which point the dose of vasopressin is incrementally decreased until no bleeding is noted after 12 hours of only saline infusion. The catheters are removed at this point.

Though catheter placement is simple from a technical standpoint, vasopressin infusion is a time-consuming procedure for the clinical teams and the

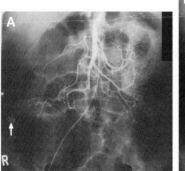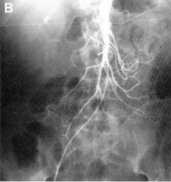

Fig. 3. A 68-year-old man with lower gastrointestinal bleeding. (A) Diagnostic angiogram of superior mesenteric artery shows a bleeding site in the cecum (*arrow*). (B) Following the infusion of 0.1 units/min of vasopressin for 20 minutes, the bleeding has ceased. Only a small amount of residual contrast remains in the bowel, but no active bleeding was noted. Note the smaller caliber of the SMA branches, demonstrating the vasoconstrictive effects of the vasopressin.

patient. The patient is often on the angiographic table for several hours and may spend up to 48 hours in an intensive care unit while the medication is being infused. Furthermore, patient cooperation is essential to prevent catheter dislodgment from the target vessel, which is surprisingly rare, occurring in less than 2% of patients in a large patient series [32].

Although vasopressin infusion is in effect treating an entire mesenteric distribution rather than the localized bleeding site, it has been shown to be an effective therapy for lower GI bleeding. Darcy recently reviewed five series with mixed lesions, including the small and large bowel, and no specific disease process and found success rates ranged from 59% to 90% overall [33]. However, success rates for colonic diverticular bleeding ranged from 92% to 100% in three different series where such specifics were stated [33]. It is not surprising, however, that rebleeding occurs in almost 40% of patients following vasopressin infusion [34,35]. The vasoconstrictive effects quickly abate once the infusion is discontinued and one relies on the patient's coagulation system to prevent further hemorrhage. Of note is that little recent work has been done on the efficacy of vasopressin infusion. Of the eight series reviewed by Darcy, as well as the referenced literature here on rebleeding, only one is less than 20 years old, that one being almost 10 years old [33]. Sherman and colleagues infused vasopressin into 71 patients, 13 of whom were treated for colonic bleeding [16]. Complete control of hemorrhage occurred in eight patients (63%). Although the complications were not divided between upper GI bleeding, including varices, from that in the lower tract, major complications occurred in 22 patients (primarily pulmonary edema and myocardial depression). Although higher than other studies, the authors note their strict criteria for citing complications and an ill patient population as contributing etiological factors.

Despite the promising success of vasopressin infusion, the interventional community has embraced transcatheter embolotherapy in recent years. Embolotherapy for lower GI bleeding was reported at almost the same time as vasopressin infusion but had an unacceptably high bowel ischemic rate and quickly fell out of favor [36]. Most believe such high rates were due to the availability of only large catheters and primitive embolic agents by today's standards. However, since the advent of microcatheters (3 French or less) and associated embolics, superselective transcatheter embolization (Fig. 4) has become the preferred technique of almost all interventionists. Last year, one of the authors was attending a workshop of approximately 100 US interventionists where an audience poll noted not a single one had infused vasopressin for lower GI bleeding in the past 2 years, whereas 100% had performed embolotherapy. Although this information is completely unscientific, it still serves to demonstrate the current attitudes of interventionists approaching lower gastrointestinal bleeding.

Transcatheter embolotherapy for the lower gastrointestinal tract is much like that described for upper GI bleeding. Usually through the catheter already in place from the diagnostic angiogram, a microcatheter and appropriately small guide wire are advanced as close to the bleeding site as possible (see Fig. 4).

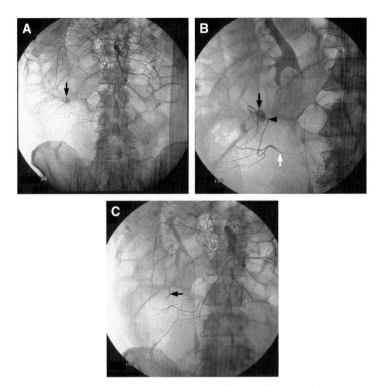

Fig. 4. A 42-year-old man with lower gastrointestinal bleeding. (A) Diagnostic angiogram of superior mesenteric artery shows a bleeding site in the right colon (*arrow*). (B) Superselective microcatheter placement demonstrates bleeding site (*arrow*). Catheter was easily advanced into the branch just at the bleeding site, and embolization with microcoils was performed. (C) Follow-up SMA angiography shows coils in place (*arrow*) and absence of hemorrhage.

Once this is confirmed with contrast injection, occlusion of the vessel is performed usually using one of three embolic agents: microcoils, polyvinyl alcohols sponge particles, or gelatin sponge particles. Most agree that a distal site at the level of the vasa recta or marginal artery should be chosen if possible. Successful cessation of the bleeding is determined by angiography through the existing diagnostic catheter (see Fig. 4) and once successful, the catheters are then removed and the patient returned to a clinical ward.

Embolotherapy has many advantages. It eliminates the prolonged catheterization times of vasopressin infusion, is free from systemic effects, and produces an immediate cessation of hemorrhage by an empirically more pleasing mechanical blockage. The procedure itself is usually regarded as technically more difficult to perform because of the superselectivity of the microcatheter and the nature of placement of the embolic agents.

As noted previously, embolotherapy is mechanically satisfying in that the bleeding site is occluded while on the angiographic table, providing empirical evidence that the patient's hemorrhaging is treated. The results of embolotherapy for the larger available studies are presented in Table 1 and demonstrate the difficulties in achieving microcatheterization for a successful embolization and the high rates of rehemorrhage, including noncessation of the original bleeding site. Many factors have been blamed for the less than stellar embolotherapy results, including location of the bleeding site and the underlying pathology. Regarding location, Peck and colleagues found for small and large bowel embolization that the jejunum and cecum have less favorable outcomes, but the patient numbers are small [37]. Evangelista and Hallisey had two patients in whom hemostasis could not be achieved despite embolotherapy, both in the cecum, but suggested it may be related to technical factors rather than location [38]. Funaki and colleagues performed 25 technically successful embolizations limited to the colon and achieved a prolonged clinical success in 22 of 27 patients given a mean follow-up of 8.7 months but a follow-up range of 1 day to 57 months [39]. Regarding the pathological entity responsible for hemorrhage, Bandi and colleagues embolized six patients with angiodysplasia and three (50%) had recurrent hemorrhage [40]. They also had unsuccessful superselective catheter placement in 27% of their patients. Khanna, in a meta-analysis of 25 publications as well as 12 patients from the authors' center, found embolization for diverticular bleeding was successful in 85% of patients [41]. In contrast, rebleeding after embolization for nondiverticular bleeding occurred in greater than 40% of patients and over a more protracted period, prompting the authors to conclude that embolization for lower GI bleeding is most effective when treating diverticular bleeding.

Although complications with embolotherapy include those of diagnostic angiography, the most feared by far has been bowel ischemia. Certainly, superselective techniques have lessened the fears and this appears to be supported

Table 1
Selected series of transcatheter embolotherapy for lower GI bleeding

Author	Year	No. of patients	No. successfully embolized (n/%)	Ischemic complications (n/%)	Rehemorrhage (n/%)
Peck[37]	1998	21	17 (81)	0 (0)	11 (52)
Evangelista[38]	2000	17	17 (100)	2 (12)	2 (13)
Luchtefeld[44]	2000	17	17 (100)	4 (24)	3 (18)
Bandi[40]	2001	48	35 (73)	6 (13)	14 (40)
Krämer[45]	2000	19	18 (95)	4 (11)	5 (22)
Funaki[39]	2001	27	25 (93)	4 (15)	5 (20)
DeBarros[46]	2002	27	23 (100)	2 (7)	5 (22)
Kuo[43]	2003	22	22 (100)	1 (7)	3 (14)
Burgess[47]	2004	15	14 (93)	6 (43)	8 (53)
Silver[48]	2005	11	10 (91)	7 (70)	1 (10)
Nicholson[49]	2005	14	14 (100)	3 (21)	2 (14)

Successfully embolized denotes catheter and embolic agents were placed. Rehemorrhage includes inability to cease hemorrhage initially.

by animal data. Chin and colleagues deposited a total of 54 microcoils into the jejunum (n = 14), ileum (n = 26), and colon (n = 14) in the porcine model and found no histological evidence of ischemia [42]. Table 1 summarizes the ischemic complications in patient series, although it includes major and minor complications. Minor ischemic complications are those limited to findings on follow-up endoscopy suggestive of ischemia but without clinical sequella. Kuo and colleagues reviewed the literature and added their 22 patients undergoing embolotherapy for lower GI bleeding since 1996, all of which used microcatheter technology and microcoils as the preferred embolic agent [43]. In this series of 144 patients, minor ischemia occurred in 7%, and infarction was not reported (0%). Most interventionists today prefer to use microcoils when possible, although optimum coil placement requires positioning of the microcatheter distally and is therefore technically more challenging.

Retrospectively, two studies have attempted to compare the efficacy of vasopressin with embolotherapy for lower GI hemorrhage. Pennoyer and colleagues reviewed 10 patients who received vasopressin infusion, one of which rehemorrhaged (10%) versus seven and two, respectively, after receiving superselective embolotherapy (29%) [35]. In a like manner, Gomes and colleagues compared nine patients undergoing vasopressin infusion with three receiving embolotherapy and found no rebleeding in either group, although the primary success was 67% for infusion versus 100% for embolotherapy [20]. The latter was true despite the absence of advanced superselective catheters, wires, and embolic agents. Unfortunately, these data are collected retrospectively, and the numbers are far too small to reach any meaningful conclusions.

SUMMARY
Diagnostic angiography still plays an essential role in the diagnosis of patients, particularly those with acute lower GI bleeding. Transcatheter therapy appears to be a viable treatment alternative in selected patients with GI bleeding. Many interventionists today believe embolotherapy to be more effective initially and to have better long-term results, specifically less rebleeding, than vasopressin infusion with at least equal complication rates. Unfortunately, direct comparison of the two techniques in a randomized, controlled fashion has not been performed. Small patient series, such as those summarized here, suggest that the results of the two techniques are essentially equal, and ischemic complications appear more prevalent with embolotherapy.

The use of embolotherapy—either empirically based on endoscopic or surgical findings or directed against a site found to have contrast extravasation—represents the current intervention of choice in the case of upper GI bleeding refractory to endoscopic intervention. Head-to-head studies directly comparing the efficacy, morbidity, and mortality associated with endovascular or surgical correction of bleeding from the upper GI tract is needed. Although the current tide favors embolotherapy in the lower GI tract, infusion of vasoconstricting agents deserves more attention. To that end, there is a great need for scientific data regarding the safety and efficacy of transcatheter therapy for upper and lower GI bleeding.

References

[1] Baum S, Nusbaum M, Blakemore WS, et al. The preoperative radiographic demonstration of intraabdominal bleeding from undetermined sites by percutaneous selective celiac and superior mesenteric arteriography. Surgery 1965;58:797.

[2] Xu ZB, Zhou XY, Peng ZY, et al. Evaluation of selective hepatic angiography and embolization in patients with massive hemobilia. Hepatobiliary Pancreat Dis Int 2005;4: 254–8.

[3] Spies JB, Bakal CW, Burke DR, et al, for the Standards of Practice Committee for the Society of Vascular and Interventional Radiology. Standard for diagnostic arteriography in adults. J Vasc Interv Radiol 1993;4:385–95.

[4] Cohn SM, Moller BA, Zieg PM, et al. Angiography for preoperative evaluation in patients with lower gastrointestinal bleeding: are the benefits worth the risks? Arch Surg 1998;133: 50–5.

[5] Aina R, Oliva V, Therasse E, et al. Arterial embolotherapy for upper gastrointestinal hemorrhage: outcome assessment. J Vasc Interv Radiol 2001;12:195–200.

[6] Schenker M, Duszak R, Soulen M, et al. Upper gastrointestinal hemorrhage and transcatheter embolotherapy: clinical and technical factors impacting success and survival. J Vasc Interv Radiol 2001;12:1263–71.

[7] Fiorito JJ, Brandt LJ, Kozicky O, et al. The diagnostic yield of superior mesenteric angiography: correlation with the pattern of gastrointestinal bleeding. Am J Gastroenterol 1989;84(8):878–81.

[8] Koval G, Benner KG, Rosch J, Kozak BE. Aggressive angiographic diagnosis in acute lower gastrointestinal hemorrhage. Dig Dis Sci 1987;32(3):248–53.

[9] Zuckerman DA, Bocchini TP. Birnbaum. Massive hemorrhage in the lower gastrointestinal tract in adults: diagnostic imaging and intervention. AJR Am J Roentgenol 1993;161: 703–11.

[10] Lieberman D. Gastrointestinal bleeding: initial management. Gastroenterol Clin North Am 1993;22:723–36.

[11] Smith R, Copely DJ, Bolen FH. ^{99m}Tc RBC Scintigraphy: correlation of gastrointestinal bleeding rates with scintigraphic findings. AJR Am J Roentgenol 1987;148:869–74.

[12] Gunderman R, Leef J, Ong K, et al. Scintigraphic screening prior to visceral arteriography in acute lower gastrointestinal bleeding. J Nucl Med 1998;39:1081–3.

[13] Malden ES, Hicks ME, Royal HD, et al. Recurrent gastrointestinal bleeding: use of thrombolysis with anticoagulation in diagnosis. Radiology 1998;207:147–51.

[14] Ryan JM, Key SM, Dumbleton SA, et al. Nonlocalized lower gastrointestinal bleeding: provocative bleeding studies with intraarterial tPA, heparin, and tolazoline. J Vasc Interv Radiol 2002;13:548–9.

[15] Barr JW, Lakin RC, Rösch J. Vasopressin and hepatic artery: effect of selective celiac infusion of vasopressin on the hepatic artery flow. Invest Radiol 1975;10:200–5.

[16] Sherman LM, Shenoy SS, Cerra FB. Selective intraarterial vasopressin: clinical efficacy and complications. Ann Surg 1979;189:298–302.

[17] Clark RA, Colley DP, Eggers FM. Acute arterial gastrointestinal hemorrhage: efficacy of transcatheter control. AJR Am J Roentgenol 1981;136:1185–9.

[18] Dahl CR, Mallory A, Hansen R, et al. Continuous intravenous vasopressin for upper gastrointestinal hemorrhage: a controlled trial [abstract]. Gastroenterology 1983;84:1132.

[19] Eckstein MR, Kelemouridis V, Athanasoulis CA, et al. Gastric bleeding: therapy with intraarterial vasopressin and transcatheter embolization. Radiology 1984;152:643–6.

[20] Gomes AS, Lois JF, McCoy RD. Angiographic treatment of gastrointestinal hemorrhage: comparison of vasopressin and embolization. AJR Am J Roentgenol 1986;146: 1031–7.

[21] Stump DL, Hardin TC. The use of vasopressin in the treatment of upper gastrointestinal hae-morrhage. Drugs 1990;39:38–53.

[22] Rosch J, Dotter CT, Brown MJ. Selective arterial embolization: a new method for control of acute gastrointestinal bleeding. Radiology 1972;102:303–6.

[23] Dempsey DT, Burke DR, Reilly RS, et al. Angiography in poor-risk patients with massive non-variceal upper gastrointestinal bleeding. Am J Surg 1990;159:282–6.

[24] Lang EV, Picus D, Marx MV, et al. Massive upper gastrointestinal hemorrhage with normal findings on arteriography: value of prophylactic embolization of the left gastric artery. AJR Am J Roentgenol 1992;158:547–9.

[25] Lang EK. Transcatheter embolization in management of hemorrhage from duodenal ulcer: long-term results and complications. Radiology 1992;182:703–7.

[26] Encarnacion CE, Kadir S, Beam CA, et al. Gastrointestinal bleeding: treatment with gastro-intestinal arterial embolization. AJR Am J Roentgenol 1992;183:505–8.

[27] Toyoda H, Nakano S, Takeda I, et al. Transcatheter arterial embolization for massive bleed-ing from duodenal ulcers not controlled by endoscopic hemostasis. Endoscopy 1995;27: 304–7.

[28] Walsh RM, Anain P, Geisinger M, et al. Role of angiography and embolization for massive gastroduodenal hemorrhage. J Gastrointest Surg 1999;3:61–5.

[29] Ripoll C, Banares R, Beceiro I, et al. Comparison of transcatheter arterial embolization and surgery for treatment of bleeding peptic ulcer after endoscopic treatment failure. J Vasc In-terv Radiol 2004;15:447–50.

[30] Lieberman DA, Keller FS, Katon RM, et al. Arterial embolization for massive upper gas-trointestinal tract bleeding in poor surgical candidates. Gastroenterology 1984;86: 876–85.

[31] Baum S, Nusbaum M. The control of gastrointestinal hemorrhage by selective mesenteric arterial infusion of vasopressin. Radiology 1971;98:497–505.

[32] Kadir S, Athanasoulis CA. Catheter dislodgement: a cause of failure of intraarterial vaso-pressin infusions to control gastrointestinal bleeding. Cardiovasc Radiol 1978;1:187–91.

[33] Darcy M. Treatment of lower gastrointestinal bleeding: vasopressin infusion versus emboli-zation. J Vasc Interv Radiol 2003;14:535–43.

[34] Johnson WC, Wildrich WC. Efficacy of selective splanchnic arteriography and vasopressin perfusion in diagnosis and treatment of gastrointestinal hemorrhage. Am J Surg 1976;131: 481–9.

[35] Pennoyer WP, Vignati PV, Cohen JL. Management of angiogram positive lower gastrointes-tinal hemorrhage: long term follow-up of non-operative treatments. Int J Colorect Dis 1996;11:279–82.

[36] Bookstein JJ, Chlosta EM, Foley D, et al. Transcatheter hemostasis of gastrointestinal bleed-ing using modified autologous clot. Radiology 1974;113:277–85.

[37] Peck DJ, McLoughlin RF, Hughson MN, et al. Percutaneous embolotherapy of lower gastro-intestinal hemorrhage. J Vasc Interv Radiol 1998;9:747–51.

[38] Evangelista PT, Hallisey MJ. Transcatheter embolization for acute lower gastrointestinal hemorrhage. J Vasc Interv Radiol 2000;11:601–6.

[39] Funaki B, Kostelic JK, Lorenz J, et al. Superselective microcoil embolization of colonic hem-orrhage. AJR 2001;177:829–36.

[40] Bandi R, Shetty PC, Sharma RP, et al. Superselective arterial embolization for the treatment of lower gastrointestinal hemorrhage. J Vasc Interv Radiol 2001;12:1399–404.

[41] Khanna A, Ognibene SJ, Koniaris LG. Embolization as the first-line therapy for diverticulosis-related massive lower gastrointestinal bleeding: evidence from a meta-analysis. J Gastroin-tenst Surg 2005;9:343–52.

[42] Chin AC, Singer MA, Mihalov M, et al. Superselective mesenteric embolization with micro-coils in a porcine model. Dis Colon Rectum 2002;45:212–8.

[43] Kuo WT, Lee DE, Saad WEA, et al. Superselective microcoil embolization for the treatment of lower gastrointestinal hemorrhage. J Vasc Interv Radiol 2003;14:1503–9.

[44] Luchtefeld MA, Senagore AJ, Szomstein M, et al. Evaluation of transarterial embolization for lower gastrointestinal bleeding. Dis Colon Rectum 2000;43:532–4.

[45] Krämer SC, Görich J, Rilinger N, et al. Embolization for gastrointestinal hemorrhages. Eur Radiol 2000;10:802–5.

[46] DeBarros J, Rosas L, Cohen J, et al. The changing paradigm for the treatment of colonic hemorrhage: superselective angiographic embolization. Dis Colon Rectum 2002;45:802–8.

[47] Burgess AN, Evans PM. Lower gastrointestinal haemorrhage and superselective angiographic embolization. ANZ J Surg 2004;74:635–8.

[48] Silver A, Bendick P, Wasvary H. Safety and efficacy of superselective angioembolization in control of lower gastrointestinal hemorrhage. Am J Surg 2005;189:361–3.

[49] Nicholson AA, Ettles DF, Hartley JE, et al. Transcatheter coil embolotherapy: a safe and effective option for major colonic haemorrhage. Gut 1998;43:79–84.

Gastroenterol Clin N Am 34 (2005) 753–775

GASTROENTEROLOGY CLINICS
OF NORTH AMERICA

CUMULATIVE INDEX 2005

Note: Page numbers of article titles are in **boldface** type.

Changing Your Address?

Make sure your subscription changes too! When you notify us of your new address, you can help make our job easier by including an exact copy of your Clinics label number with your old address (see illustration below.) This number identifies you to our computer system and will speed the processing of your address change. Please be sure this label number accompanies your old address and your corrected address—you can send an old Clinics label with your number on it or just copy it exactly and send it to the address listed below.

We appreciate your help in our attempt to give you continuous coverage. Thank you.

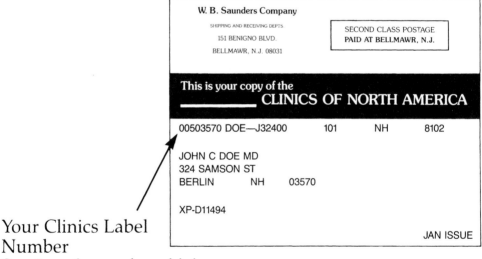

Your Clinics Label Number

Copy it exactly or send your label along with your address to:
W.B. Saunders Company, Customer Service
Orlando, FL 32887-4800
Call Toll Free 1-800-654-2452

Please allow four to six weeks for delivery of new subscriptions and for processing address changes.

United States Postal Service
Statement of Ownership, Management, and Circulation

1. Publication Title	2. Publication Number									3. Filing Date
Gastroenterology Clinics of North America	0	8	8	9	-	8	5	5	3	9/15/05

4. Issue Frequency	5. Number of Issues Published Annually	6. Annual Subscription Price
Mar, Jun, Sep, Dec	4	$190.00

7. Complete Mailing Address of Known Office of Publication *(Not printer)* *(Street, city, county, state, and ZIP+4)*

Elsevier Inc.
6277 Sea Harbor Drive
Orlando, FL 32887-4800

Contact Person
Gwen C. Campbell
Telephone
215-239-3685

8. Complete Mailing Address of Headquarters or General Business Office of Publisher *(Not printer)*

Elsevier Inc., 360 Park Avenue South, New York, NY 10010-1710

9. Full Names and Complete Mailing Addresses of Publisher, Editor, and Managing Editor *(Do not leave blank)*
Publisher *(Name and complete mailing address)*

Tim Griswold, Elsevier Inc., 1600 John F. Kennedy Blvd., Suite 1800, Philadelphia, PA 19103-2899
Editor *(Name and complete mailing address)*

Carin Davis, Elsevier Inc., 1600 John F. Kennedy Blvd., Suite 1800, Philadelphia, PA 19103-2899
Managing Editor *(Name and complete mailing address)*

Heather Cullen, Elsevier Inc., 1600 John F. Kennedy Blvd., Suite 1800, Philadelphia, PA 19103-2899

10. Owner *(Do not leave blank. If the publication is owned by a corporation, give the name and address of the corporation immediately followed by the names and addresses of all stockholders owning or holding 1 percent or more of the total amount of stock. If not owned by a corporation, give the names and addresses of the individual owners. If owned by a partnership or other unincorporated firm, give its name and address as well as those of each individual owner. If the publication is published by a nonprofit organization, give its name and address.)*

Full Name	Complete Mailing Address
Wholly owned subsidiary of	4520 East-West Highway
Reed/Elsevier Inc., US holdings	Bethesda, MD 20814

11. Known Bondholders, Mortgagees, and Other Security Holders Owning or
Holding 1 Percent or More of Total Amount of Bonds, Mortgages, or
Other Securities. If none, check box ▸ ☐ None

Full Name	Complete Mailing Address
N/A	

12. Tax Status *(For completion by nonprofit organizations authorized to mail at nonprofit rates)* *(Check one)*
The purpose, function, and nonprofit status of this organization and the exempt status for federal income tax purposes:
☐ Has Not Changed During Preceding 12 Months
☐ Has Changed During Preceding 12 Months *(Publisher must submit explanation of change with this statement)*

(See Instructions on Reverse)

PS Form **3526**, October 1999

13. Publication Title	14. Issue Date for Circulation Data Below
Gastroenterology Clinics of North America	June 2005

15.	Extent and Nature of Circulation		Average No. Copies Each Issue During Preceding 12 Months	No. Copies of Single Issue Published Nearest to Filing Date
a.	Total Number of Copies *(Net press run)*		3400	3200
b. Paid and/or Requested Circulation	(1)	Paid/Requested Outside-County Mail Subscriptions Stated on Form 3541. *(Include advertiser's proof and exchange copies)*	1632	1525
	(2)	Paid In-County Subscriptions Stated on Form 3541 *(Include advertiser's proof and exchange copies)*		
	(3)	Sales Through Dealers and Carriers, Street Vendors, Counter Sales, and Other Non-USPS Paid Distribution	794	731
	(4)	Other Classes Mailed Through the USPS		
c.	Total Paid and/or Requested Circulation *[Sum of 15b. (1), (2), (3), and (4)]* ▸		2426	2256
d. Free Distribution by Mail *(Samples, compliment-ary, and other free)*	(1)	Outside-County as Stated on Form 3541	97	109
	(2)	In-County as Stated on Form 3541		
	(3)	Other Classes Mailed Through the USPS		
e.	Free Distribution Outside the Mail *(Carriers or other means)*			
f.	Total Free Distribution *(Sum of 15d. and 15e.)* ▸		97	109
g.	Total Distribution *(Sum of 15c. and 15f.)* ▸		2523	2365
h.	Copies not Distributed		877	835
i.	Total *(Sum of 15g. and h.)* ▸		3400	3200
j.	Percent Paid and/or Requested Circulation *(15c. divided by 15g. times 100)*		96%	95%

16. Publication of Statement of Ownership
☐ Publication required. Will be printed in the **December 2005** issue of this publication.
☐ Publication not required.

17. Signature and Title of Editor, Publisher, Business Manager, or Owner

[signature]
John Panucci – Executive Director of Subscription Services

Date
9/15/05

I certify that all information furnished on this form is true and complete. I understand that anyone who furnishes false or misleading information on this form or who omits material or information requested on the form may be subject to criminal sanctions (including fines and imprisonment) and/or civil sanctions (including civil penalties).

Instructions to Publishers

1. Complete and file one copy of this form with your postmaster annually on or before October 1. Keep a copy of the completed form for your records.
2. In cases where the stockholder or security holder is a trustee, include in items 10 and 11 the name of the person or corporation for whom the trustee is acting. Also include the names and addresses of individuals who are stockholders who own or hold 1 percent or more of the total amount of bonds, mortgages, or other securities of the publishing corporation. In item 11, if none, check the box. Use blank sheets if more space is required.
3. Be sure to furnish all circulation information called for in item 15. Free circulation must be shown in items 15d, e, and f.
4. Item 15h., Copies not Distributed, must include (1) newsstand copies originally stated on Form 3541, and returned to the publisher, (2) estimated returns from news agents, and (3), copies for office use, leftovers, spoiled, and all other copies not distributed.
5. If the publication had Periodicals authorization as a general or requester publication, this Statement of Ownership, Management, and Circulation must be published; it must be printed in any issue in October or, if the publication is not published during October, the first issue printed after October.
6. In item 16, indicate the date of the issue in which this Statement of Ownership will be published.
7. Item 17 must be signed.
Failure to file or publish a statement of ownership may lead to suspension of Periodicals authorization.

PS Form **3526**, October 1999 *(Reverse)*